Clinical Paediatric Haematology and Oncology

Clinical Paediatric Haematology and Oncology

EDITED BY

HENRY EKERT
MD FRACP FRCPA
Director, Department of
Clinical Haematology and Oncology,
Royal Children's Hospital, Melbourne

Blackwell Scientific Publications
MELBOURNE OXFORD LONDON
EDINBURGH BOSTON

Editorial offices:
99 Barry Street, Carlton
Victoria 3053, Australia
Osney Mead, Oxford OX2 OEL
8 John Street, London WC1N 2ES
9 Forrest Road, Edinburgh EH1 2QH
52 Beacon Street, Boston
Massachusetts 02108, USA

First published 1982

Typeset by ABB Typesetting Pty Ltd

Printed in Australia by Brown Prior Anderson Pty Ltd Burwood Victoria

DISTRIBUTORS

USA
Blackwell Mosby Book Distributors
11830 Westline Industrial Drive
St Louis, Missouri 63141

Canada
Blackwell Mosby Book Distributors
120 Melford Drive, Scaborough
Ontario M1B 2X4

Australia
Blackwell Scientific Book
Distributors
214 Berkeley Street, Carlton
Victoria 3053

Cataloguing in Publication Data
Clinical paediatric haematology and oncology.

Bibliography.
Includes index.
ISBN 0 86793 000 4.

1. Pediatric hematology.
2. Tumors in children.
I. Ekert, Henry.

618.92'15

Contents

Contributors

NEIL T. CAMPBELL FRACP
Director, Department of Neonatology, Royal Children's Hospital, Melbourne
Chapter 15

HENRY EKERT MD FRACP FRCPA
Director, Department of Clinical Haematology and Oncology, Royal Children's Hospital, Melbourne
Chapters 1–7 and, in collaboration, Chapters 16–23

CLIFFORD S. HOSKING MD FRACP FRCPA
Director, Department of Immunology, Royal Children's Hospital, Melbourne
Chapter 8

RAE N. MATTHEWS MRCP FRACP DCH
Associate Clinical Haematologist, Royal Children's Hospital, Melbourne
Chapters 13, 14 and, in collaboration, Chapter 15

GEOFFREY P. TAURO FRACP FRCPA
Director Haematology Laboratory, Royal Children's Hospital, Melbourne
Chapters 9–12

KEITH D. WATERS FRACP
Deputy Director, Department of Clinical Haematology and Oncology, Royal Children's Hospital, Melbourne
Chapters 16–23

Preface

This book has been written to provide an overview of the practice of clinical haematology and oncology as it occurs in specialized units within general paediatric teaching hospitals. The text reflects a practical approach to the problems encountered in the wards and outpatient clinics. Whenever possible, attempts have been made to integrate pertinent physiology, pathology, clinical features and management into a short pertinent unit which can be applied to clinical management. The text does not aim to comprehensively cover basic physiology, biochemistry and pathology, nor are there attempts to debate obscure or currently unsolved problems in haematology and oncology. In order to keep the book at a reasonable size, rare haematological and oncological conditions have been omitted. These are already well described in more specialized texts on haematology or oncology.

The authors hope that the book will prove particularly useful to medical students and junior medical officers who work in haematology and oncology units, as well as trainees who intend to specialize in haematology and oncology. For the latter group, the book may act as an introduction prior to consulting more detailed texts. Hopefully, some of the views expressed in this book will stimulate the reader to debate and personal research.

It is hoped that this book will also prove particularly useful for members of medical allied professions who work in or with haematology and oncology units. The comprehensive text books on haematology and oncology are too detailed and theoretical to be of much value to these professions. In this book, we have attempted to provide information which will highlight some of the problems involved in medical management, and to bring the reader up-to-date with current results of treatment and an understanding of the nature of the disease process.

In order to reduce long lists of footnotes and references, statements of fact or theory have not been referenced in the text, but rather a recommended reading list has been provided for each chapter. In this sense, the book serves as an introduction to the subject of haematology and oncology. These lists substantiate the point of view described by the authors, but are clearly not meant as a comprehensive literature review, which, in any case, becomes rapidly dated.

I am indebted to many for the production of this book. My particular thanks are extended to members of staff of my unit and the hospital, who not only contributed to this book but also endured the increased work load and strain entailed in its writing. I am grateful to Mr Peter Jones for encouraging me to undertake the task, and to my wife and family for bearing with me.

Particular thanks are extended to my secretary, Mrs Margaret Cameron, without whose excellent work on the collection and typing of the manuscript, as well as arrangement of diagrams, this book would not have been possible.

Melbourne 1982 Henry Ekert

Chapter 1 The Physiology of Haemostasis

Definition

Haemostasis is that series of physiological processes which arrest bleeding at the site of injury and initiate repair of the blood vessel. Haemostasis involves three main components: (1) blood vessels, (2) platelets, (3) the coagulation and fibrinolytic enzymes.

There is much detailed knowledge of platelets, coagulation and fibrinolysis. On the other hand, investigations of the role of endothelium, subendothelium and collagen are still preliminary.

INTERACTION OF PLATELETS AND BLOOD VESSELS

Injury to the blood vessel is associated with damage to the endothelium and exposure of subendothelium and, in more severe vessel injury, collagen. Platelets can adhere to the subendothelial matrix and collagen. Adhesion to the subendothelial matrix requires the presence of a functional part of the factor VIII complex, known as the von Willebrand factor. Components of factor VIII are synthesized in endothelial cells and may be released from the cells when there is vessel injury.

Adhesion of platelets is followed by their aggregation (Fig. 1.1). The process of aggregation is mediated by the release of stored materials in the dense granules of the platelets, the principal one being adenosine diphosphate (ADP). The process of storage of ADP in the dense granules and its release require normal platelet metabolism. The release process appears to be mediated by activation of the enzyme phospholipase which produces arachidonic acid from platelet membrane phospholipid. Arachidonic acid is oxidized by cyclo-oxygenase to form prostaglandin intermediates and thromboxane A_2 which greatly promotes platelet aggregation through the release reaction. Thromboxane A_2 is rapidly oxidized to thromboxane B which does not promote platelet aggregation. The process is diagrammatically summarized in Fig. 1.2. Platelet aggregation resulting from thromboxane A_2 synthesis is associated with a decrease of cyclic AMP and an increase of calcium levels in the platelet. These changes are associated with release of the platelet non-metabolic pool of ADP and aggregation of the platelets. For platelet aggregation to occur, there must be receptors for ADP on the platelet membrane. The exact mechanism whereby the reaction of

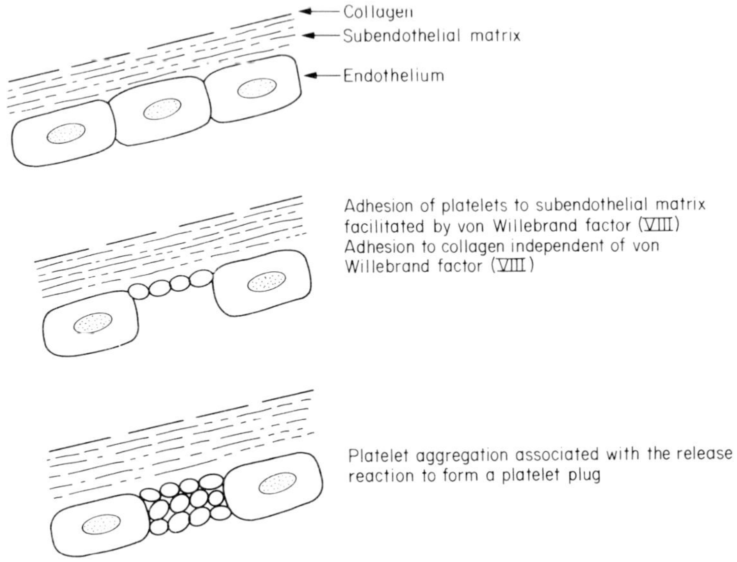

Fig. 1.1 Platelet adhesion and aggregation.

ADP with the platelet membrane receptor causes aggregation of platelets remains speculative. Abnormalities of platelet adhesion and aggregation are generally associated with bruising and mucosal bleeding, and the laboratory findings of a prolonged bleeding time.

Endothelial cells can react with the prostaglandin intermediates synthesized in the platelets to form prostacyclins, and recently it has been shown that prostacyclins can also be produced in the platelets (Fig. 1.2). These substances actively inhibit platelet aggregation. It is possible, but not proven, that a balance between thromboxane A_2 and prostacyclin synthesis may regulate the size and spread of the platelet aggregate that follows vessel injury.

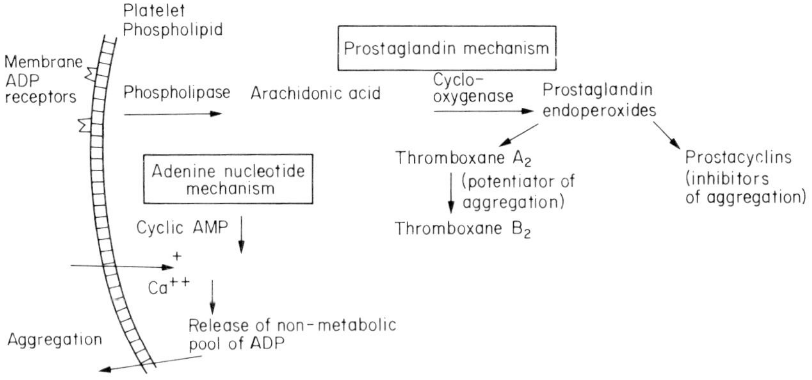

Fig. 1.2 Key processes involved in platelet aggregation.

PLATELET COAGULANT ACTIVITIES

It is now well established that platelets contribute procoagulant activities which can accelerate the process of coagulation and possibly localize it to the surface of the platelet aggregate. The platelet surface membrane phospholipids are required for rapid conversion of certain procoagulants (factor X and II) to active enzymes. Platelets may also release particles which act as general procoagulants. These combined activities are known as platelet factor 3 (PF_3). The release reaction is also associated with the appearance of an antiheparin activity known as platelet factor 4 (PF_4), a protein of unknown functional activity and structural similarity to PF_4, known as β-thromboglobulin, antiplasmin activity and antiplasminogen activator activity. In addition, there is good evidence that platelets can release procoagulant activities which have the characteristics of activated factors XI and V. The precise role and sequence in which these platelet procoagulant activities interact to secure haemostasis is unknown at present.

PLASMA COAGULANT ACTIVITIES

A scheme illustrating an acceptable current concept of procoagulant enzyme interactions is shown in Fig. 1.3. It is now considered that factor XII (Hageman factor) plays a more important role in interactions with the fibrinolytic mechanism, the complement system and vasoactive kinins than in coagulation (Fig. 1.4). Factor VIII and V appear to act as rate limiting substances in the conversion of X → Xa and II (prothrombin) to IIa (thrombin) respectively. It is considered that the role of the intrinsic coagulation system is to amplify the coagulation response to vessel injury. The trigger for this amplification may be the generation of trace amounts of thrombin from the extrinsic pathway. Thrombin also acts to activate factor XIII which crosslinks fibrin by transamidation between Σ-amino group of lysine and γ-amide group of glutamine. The coagulation pathway can be summarized as shown in Fig. 1.5.

A combination of two screening tests of the coagulation pathway may give information as to the possible site of the coagulation disorder. The activated partial thromboplastin time (APTT) tests the integrity of the intrinsic and common pathways. The one stage prothrombin time (PT) tests the integrity of the extrinsic and common pathways. Thus, a prolonged APTT and normal PT indicate an intrinsic pathway defect, prolonged PT and normal APTT an extrinsic defect; prolonged PT and PTT on an adequate blood sample are most often due to disseminated intravascular coagulation or congenital defects of the common pathway.

Activated coagulation factors can be inactivated by naturally occurring plasma proteins of which antithrombin III (α_2-ATIII) is the most important. ATIII inhibits the serine protease activity of thrombin and activated coagulation factors Xa, IXa, XIa and possibly XIIa. The rate and amount of

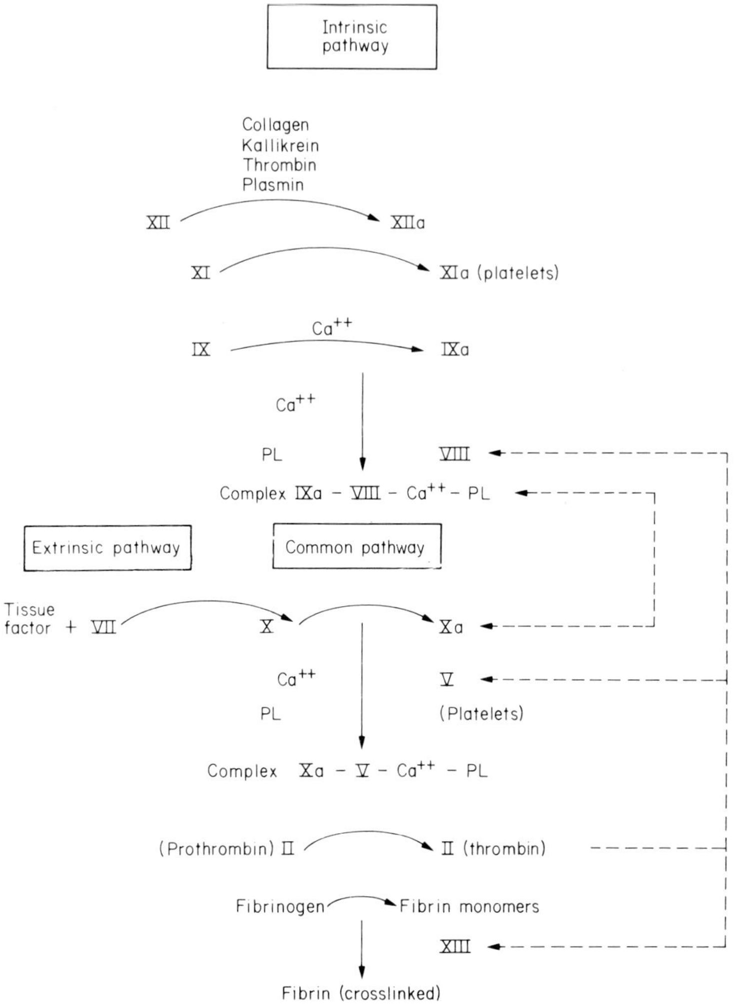

Fig. 1.3 A scheme of the mechanism of blood coagulation. PL: Phospholipid. Broken lines indicate that thrombin or Xa accelerated the reaction.

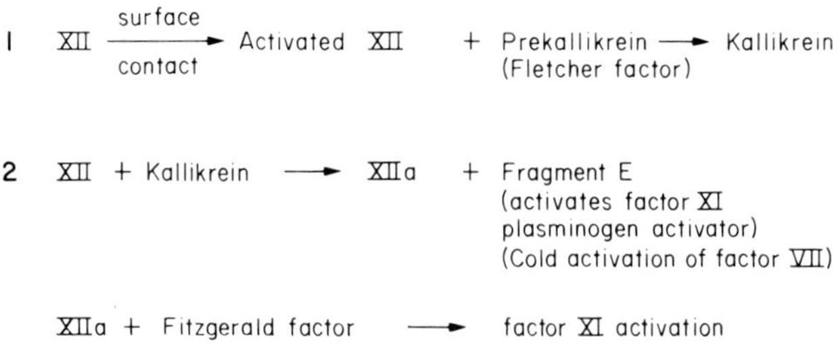

Fig. 1.4 Interaction of factor XII with the fibrinolytic mechanism, the complement system and vasoactive kinins.

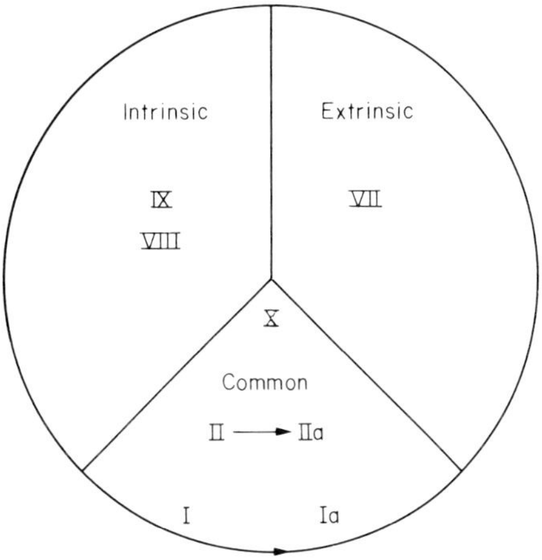

Fig. 1.5 Summary of coagulation pathway.

inactivation of Xa is increased by heparin. Heparin also increases the rate of inactivation of thrombin and XIa, but has little effect on the amount inactivated. Potentiation of ATIII activity by low doses of heparin is considered to be the explanation for the effectiveness of prophylactic low dose heparin in prevention of venous thrombosis.

FIBRINOLYSIS

The fibrinolytic system is based on the activation of a zymogen (plasminogen) to a serine protease plasmin (Fig. 1.6). Plasminogen is present in plasma and is closely associated with fibrinogen. The conversion of plasminogen to plasmin requires the presence of tissue activators which are widely distributed, being

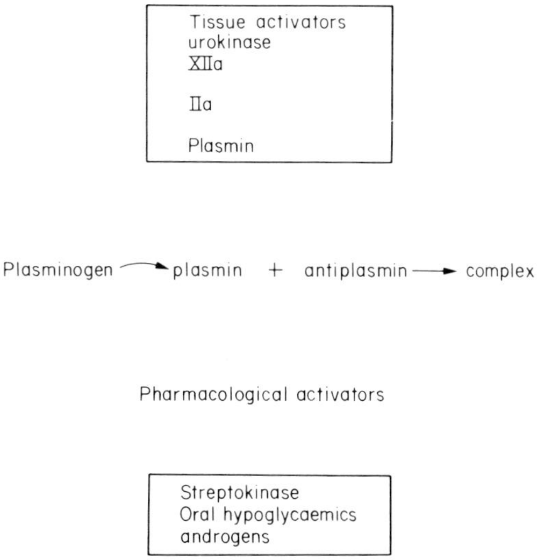

Fig. 1.6 Naturally occurring activators.

present in endothelium and cells of tissues such as lung and uterus. Urokinase which is synthesized in the kidney is an activator recovered from the urine and available in a highly purified form. The mechanism of activation of plasminogen by plasma factors is complicated and has not yet been fully worked out. Plasminogen can be activated by activation of factor XII in the presence of kallikrein, but activators not dependent on factor XII have also been described.

Under normal circumstances, plasmin forms a complex with its inhibitor antiplasmin (α_2-macroglobulin and α_1-antiplasmin) so that there is no free fibrinolytic activity. α_2-macroglobulin has some weak antithrombin and anti-Xa activity, while antithrombin III has weak antiplasmin activity. Inhibitors of plasminogen activators are present in platelets and may be of importance in inhibiting plasmin activity within a haemostatic plug.

The mechanisms whereby plasmin causes dissolution of a thrombus are not fully understood. There are three favoured theories which are not mutually exclusive:

1 Diffusion of activators from damaged endothelium may set up a localized fibrinolytic process.

2 Diffusion of plasmin bound to antiplasmin may occur from plasma to thrombus because of the greater affinity of plasmin for fibrin than antiplasmin.

3 Perfusion of the thrombus by circulating plasminogen may result in the activation of the plasminogen by tissue activators in the thrombus.

Plasmin digestion of fibrinogen and fibrin takes place as an orderly sequence. First, large molecular weight breakdown products appear with immunological characteristics similar to the protein of origin. The initial high molecular weight degradation product of fibrinogen or fibrin is called X and is due, principally, to digestion of the α chain of fibrinogen. Its further degradation by plasmin in the case of fibrinogen liberates a smaller molecular weight product with a distinct antigenic site called D, which is a disulphide linked portion of β and γ chains, and the remainder of the degraded now asymmetric molecule is called Y and retains the antigenic properties of the parent molecule. Further digestion of Y leads to two distinct end products of digestion, another molecule of D and a smaller molecular weight product E consisting of disulphide linked *N*-terminal portions of α, β and γ chains. In the case of crosslinked fibrin plasmin digestion proceeds to produce the product X, E and dimers of D (D–D). The scheme of fibrinogen lysis is outlined in Fig. 1.7.

Fibrinogen/fibrin degradation products can act as anticoagulants by absorbing thrombin; interfering with fibrin polymerization and probably with the process of platelet aggregation.

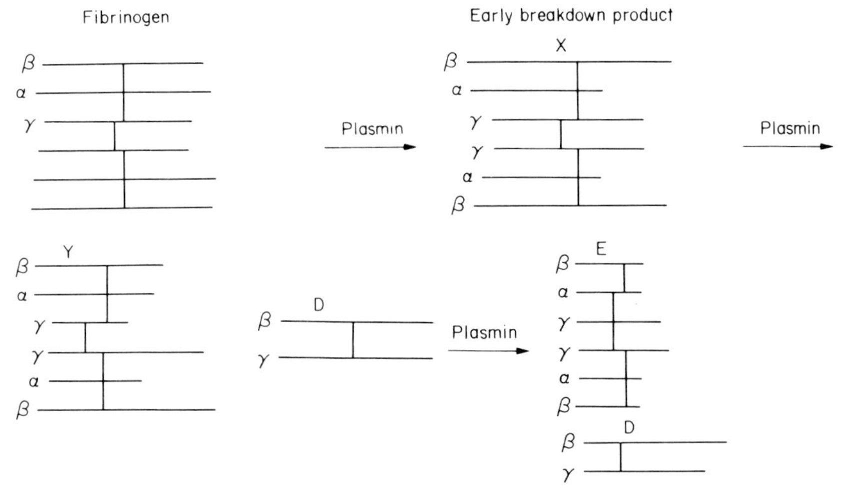

Fig. 1.7 Schematic representation of degradation of fibrinogen by plasmin. Fibrinogen is composed by α, β and γ chains held together by interchain disulphide bonds. Cleavage of predominantly the α chain results in the formation of the large MW (X) breakdown product. Further digestion results in cleavage of β + α polypeptides which are linked by interchain disulphide bond(s) and constitute fragment D. The asymmetric remaining molecule is fragment Y which is further degraded to D and a residual portion linked by *N*-terminal disulphide bonds, fragment E.

RECOMMENDED READING

CHESTERMAN C.N. (1975) The fibrinolytic system and haemostasis. *Thrombosis Diathes. Haemorrhagica* **34**, 368.

DAVIE E.W & FUJIKAWA K. (1975) Basic mechanisms in blood coagulation. *Annual Reviews, Biochemistry* **44**, 799.

GAFFNEY P.J. (1977) Structure of fibrinogen and degradation products of fibrinogen and fibrin. *British Medical Bulletin* **33**, 245.

MONCANDA S. & VANE J.R. (1979) Arachidonic acid, metabolites and the interactions between platelets and blood-vessel walls. *New England Journal of Medicine* **300**, 1142.

MUSTARD F.J. & PACKHAM M.A. (1970) Factors influencing platelet function: adhesion, release and aggregation. *Pharmacological reviews* **22**, 97.

WEISS H.J. (1975) Platelet physiology and abnormalities of platelet function. *New England Journal of Medicine* **293**, 531, 580.

Chapter 2
Investigations of Patients with Suspected Congenital Bleeding Disorders

HISTORY TAKING

Family history

A detailed family history of a bleeding tendency may give an excellent clue to the type of investigations which may most readily establish the diagnosis of the bleeding disorder. Haemophilia and Christmas disease are the most common sex-linked disorders of haemostasis and a family history which shows that males were predominantly affected or that there were unexplained deaths of male infants, suggests sex-linked inheritance. Sometimes with sex-linked inheritance, the family history of bleeding may skip generations when unaffected males were born. In the case of the above type of family history, investigations should be directed at the diagnosis of haemophilia or Christmas disease.

Von Willebrand's syndrome is the second most common disorder of haemostasis. It is usually inherited as an autosomal dominant disorder. Both sexes can be affected and frequently there is a history of bleeding in successive generations. The remainder of the congenital disorders of haemostasis are usually inherited in an autosomal recessive manner. The inheritance pattern of congenital bleeding disorders is summarized in Tables 2.1 and 2.2.

Table 2.1 Inheritance and presenting symptoms in the most common bleeding disorders.

Disease	Inheritance	Most common presenting symptoms
Haemophilia	Sex-linked	Bleeding post-circumcision, mouth trauma, haemarthroses
Christmas disease	Sex-linked	As above
Von Willebrand's syndrome	Autosomal dominant	Epistaxis and excessive bruising, unexpected postoperative haemorrhage
Congenital disorders of platelet function	Autosomal recessive occasionally dominant	As above

Table 2.2 Inheritance and presenting symptoms of rare bleeding disorders.

Disease	Inheritance	Most common presenting symptoms
Factor XI deficiency	Autosomal recessive	None or post-traumatic bleeding, spontaneous bruising, particularly in females
Factor VII deficiency	Autosomal recessive intermediate penetrance	Haemorrhage in newborn period (gastro-intestinal, cord, cerebral), gum bleeding, haemarthroses
Factor XIII	Autosomal recessive	Haemorrhage in newborn period characteristically from umbilical cord. Muscle haematomas
Factor V deficiency	Autosomal recessive ? dominant	Haemarthroses, mouth bleeding, epistaxis
Combined V and VIII deficiency	Autosomal recessive	Bruising, haematuria, bleeding after dental extraction
Factor X deficiency	Autosomal recessive	Easy bruising, epistaxis
Factor II deficiency	Autosomal recessive	Easy bruising, post-traumatic bleeding, epistaxis
Factor I deficiency hypo- and dysfibrino-genaemias	Autosomal recessive	None, post-traumatic bleeding, tendency to recurrent thromboses

GROUPING OF PATIENTS FOR INVESTIGATION

1 History of clinically significant bleeding with family history suggestive of a sex-linked disorder. The activated partial thromboplastin time is prolonged and the prothrombin time is normal. Haemophilia is the most likely diagnosis and can be confirmed by a factor VIII assay. If the factor VIII level is normal, then a factor IX assay may be performed to diagnose Christmas disease.

2 History of clinically significant bleeding with family history suggestive of autosomal dominant inheritance. Von Willebrand's syndrome is the most likely diagnosis. The investigations required to establish it are outlined below (Table 2.3).

3 History of clinically significant bleeding tendency but no family history of bleeding. Although haemophilia is the most likely diagnosis, there are other significant possibilities and in order to diminish the number of venepunctures that may be required to establish the diagnosis, sufficient blood should be sent for screening investigations and specific coagulation factor assays and a bleeding time (BT) should be performed.

Table 2.3 Results of screening tests of coagulation and platelet function in the more common congenital bleeding disorders.

Disease	APTT	PT	BT	Platelet Function: ADP	Platelet Function: Collagen	Platelet Function: Adrenalin	Platelet Function: Ristocetin	Specific confirmation
Haemophilia Christmas disease Factor XI deficiency	Prolonged	N	N	N	N	N	N	Specific factor assay
Von Willebrand's syndrome	Usually normal	N	Usually prolonged	N	N	N	Usually abnormal	Low levels of Von Willebrand factor (ristocetin cofactor)
Thrombasthenia	N	N	Prolonged	Absent	Absent	Absent	N	Normal uptake of C^{14} serotonin. Release of C^{14} serotonin (or storage pool ADP) by thrombin or collagen is normal, but absent with ADP
'Aspirin-like defect'	N	N	Prolonged	Normal at high conc. Primary only at low conc.	Absent	Absent	N	Normal uptake of C^{14} serotonin. Abnormal release with all agents. Normal storage pool of ADP

				Platelet Function				
Disease	APTT	PT	BT	ADP	Collagen	Adrenalin	Ristocetin	Specific confirmation
'Storage pool defect'	N	N	Prolonged	Normal at high conc. Primary only at low conc.	Absent	Absent	N	Abnormal uptake and release of C^{14} serotonin. Reduced or absent storage pool of ADP
Bernard-Soulier syndrome	N	N	Prolonged	N	N	N	Reduced or absent	Giant platelets, thrombocytopenia. Normal von Willebrand factor
Factor VII deficiency	N	Prolonged	Normal occasionally prolonged	N	N	N	N	Specific factor assay
Factor XIII deficiency	N	N	N	N	N	N	N	Clot dissolves in urea. Low specific assay for factor XIII
Factors X, II, V, I	Prolonged	Prolonged	N	N	N	N	N	Specific assay

Type of bleeding

The type of bleeding may also give a clue to the likely diagnosis. In haemophilia and Christmas disease, there is frequently bleeding after circumcision or after minor mouth trauma. Bruising is often more marked than in a normal child and is present on thighs, upper arms or trunk. It is uncommon for children to initially present with haemarthroses. In von Willebrand's syndrome and congenital disorders of platelet function, nose bleeding, excessive bruising or unexpected postoperative bleeding are the most common presenting features. The usual modes of presentation of the most common congenital bleeding disorders are shown in Table 2.1, and of the rare congenital bleeding disorders in Table 2.2.

Physical examination

Apart from confirming the presence of excessive bruising in regions of the body where bruising does not normally occur, physical examination of the patients is usually of little value in establishing a diagnosis.

Laboratory investigations

On the basis of a complete clinical history and the fact that the most common congenital disorders of haemostasis are haemophilia, von Willebrand's disease, Christmas disease and congenital platelet function abnormalities, laboratory investigations may be considered in the groups to be outlined. Before undertaking laboratory investigations, it should be ascertained that the patient has not taken aspirin for at least 7 days, as it can interfere with these investigations. Usual screening investigations are: (1) activated partial thromboplastin time (APTT), (2) prothrombin time (PT) and (3) template bleeding time (BT).

Further specific investigations will depend on the results of the screening tests. The following possibilities may occur:

1 PROLONGED APTT, NORMAL PT AND BT

Inspection of Fig. 1.5 shows that intrinsic pathway defects, which are most commonly haemophilia and Christmas disease, are responsible for this set of laboratory abnormalities. The diagnosis is confirmed by specific assays of factors VIII or IX.

2 PROLONGED APTT, NORMAL PT, PROLONGED BT

Von Willebrand's syndrome is characterized by abnormalities of factor VIII and a prolonged BT. The diagnosis may be confirmed by assaying the specific functional properties of the factor VIII molecule (Chapter 3). Whenever possible, the laboratory should be requested to assay factor VIII procoagulant activity; factor VIII related antigen; and von Willebrand factor (sometimes called ristocetin-cofactor), or if this is not possible, the rate of ristocetin induced platelet aggregation. The relationship of the functional and immunological properties of factor VIII are described in Chapter 3.

3 NORMAL APTT, NORMAL PT, PROLONGED BT

The most common causes of these laboratory findings are von Willebrand's syndrome and congenital platelet function abnormalities (it is assumed that ingestion of drugs that interfere with platelet function has been excluded as a cause of prolonged BT). The investigations for von Willebrand's syndrome have been outlined. They are more difficult to perform than platelet function studies. In addition, platelet function studies must be done on fresh platelet rich plasma. For these reasons, unless there is a specific family history of von Willebrand's syndrome, platelet function studies should be performed first and, if they are negative, then investigations for von Willebrand's syndrome should be pursued.

The most commonly performed investigations of platelet function are:

(a) *Platelet aggregation with ADP* This measures the ability of the platelet to aggregate in response to pharmacologic concentration of an agent that, after attachment to the platelet membrane receptor, causes platelet aggregation irrespective of the release reaction. In critical small doses, aggregation with ADP also measures the platelet release reaction as, under these circumstances, maintenance of platelet aggregation depends upon the release of platelet stores of ADP. Absent aggregation, even in the presence of high levels of ADP, is characteristic of Glanzmann's disease (thrombasthenia). Platelet release abnormalities show normal aggregation in response to high concentrations of ADP, but only a primary phase with disaggregation in response to low concentrations.

(b) *Platelet aggregation with collagen* This depends upon the ability of the platelet to adhere to collagen and to release the contents of the platelet storage granules and, in particular, stored ADP. It is abnormal in patients with platelet release abnormalities and thrombasthenia. The test is not always readily reproducible and laboratory artefacts may make results difficult to interpret.

(c) *Platelet aggregation with adrenalin* This consists of a primary reversible phase of platelet aggregation followed by the release reaction. It is a more sensitive measure of the ability of platelets to release stored ADP than the collagen test. It is abnormal in thrombasthenia and platelet release abnormalities.

(d) *Platelet aggregation with ristocetin* This depends on the presence of a normal functional activity of the factor VIII molecule independent of its procoagulant activity and on the presence of normal receptor sites (different from ADP) on the platelet membrane. Ristocetin aggregation is reduced or absent in most patients with severe von Willebrand's syndrome and in patients with the Bernard-Soulier syndrome, which is inherited as an autosomal recessive disorder and is also characterized by thrombocytopenia and a high percentage of giant platelets.

4 NORMAL APTT, PROLONGED PT, NORMAL BT

Inspection of Fig. 1.5 will show that this condition occurs only if there are abnormalities of factor VII. The condition is confirmed by specific assays of factor VII.

5 NORMAL APTT, NORMAL PT, NORMAL BT

In the absence of a family history of bleeding or significant bleeding symptoms in the patient, no further investigations are required and the patient and family may be reassured that there is no congenital bleeding tendency. In the presence of a family history or significant bleeding symptoms, detailed investigations for mild haemophilia, von Willebrand's disease or Christmas disease, should be pursued. Factor VIII or IX procoagulant levels above 20% are usually associated with a normal APTT. Mild von Willebrand's syndrome may only be diagnosed by low levels of von Willebrand factor. When all the investigations for the above disorders are normal, the possibility of congenital factor XIII deficiency should be excluded by performing screening tests for this factor. The test consists of incubating the patient's plasma clot in urea or monocloracetic acid. In the absence of factor XIII, crosslinking of fibrin monomers by covalent bonds does not occur (Fig. 1.3). The fibrin monomers are only held together by noncovalent bonds which dissociate in the above solutions.

In patients with recurrent nose bleeds and/or unexplained iron deficiency anaemia, the possibility of hereditary haemorrhagic telangiectasia should be considered. The patient should be carefully inspected for the presence of slightly raised spots consisting of dilated and tortuous vessels which bland on pressure. These are usually most obvious on the face (eyelids and lips) and/or the exposed parts of arms and thorax. Occasionally, endoscopic investigations may be required to confirm the presence of telangiectasia.

Despite detailed investigations, there still remains an ill-defined group of disorders with a definite clinical bleeding tendency but no specific laboratory abnormality. It is better to concede the fact that no label can be attached to these patients rather than label them with names such as 'purpura simplex'. The patients must be warned that they may bleed after trauma and surgery and that their bleeding may be exacerbated by the ingestion of aspirin.

6 PROLONGED APTT, PROLONGED PT, NORMAL BT

This is a rare circumstance. In the author's experience, it is most often due to a faulty collection of blood with clotting in the syringe or test-tube, or insufficient blood for the amount of anti-coagulant in the test-tube. If these artefacts have been excluded, then the most likely abnormality lies in the common pathway (Fig. 1.5). Specific assays will be required to characterize the defect. The most common congenital abnormality is dysfibrinogenemia.

A summary of the results of screening tests of coagulation and platelet function in the more common congenital bleeding disorders is shown in Table 2.3.

RECOMMENDED READING

BIGGS R. (1978) *The Treatment of Haemophilia A and B and von Willebrand's Disease.* Blackwell Scientific Publications, Oxford.

HARDISTY R.M. & INGRAM G.I.C. (1978) *Bleeding Disorders: Investigation and Management.* Blackwell Scientific Publications, Oxford.

Chapter 3
Common Congenital Disorders of Haemostasis

As haemophilia is the commonest bleeding disorder and principles of management are similar for other bleeding disorders, details of treatment will be described in the section on haemophilia, and variations from this pattern will be outlined in the appropriate sections.

HAEMOPHILIA

This is inherited as a sex-linked recessive disorder and is estimated to involve $4.5–10 \times 10^{-5}$ of the population. The presenting clinical features and the laboratory diagnosis have been described in Chapter 2.

An understanding of current knowledge of the molecular nature of factor VIII is required to permit rational management of the disorder.

Structure and functional properties of factor VIII

Factor VIII is a molecular complex with distinct functional and antigenic properties.

FUNCTIONAL PROPERTIES

1 Procoagulant activity required for activation of factor X (see Fig. 1.3); decreased or absent in haemophilia.

2 The activity required for adhesion of platelets to the subendothelial matrix and for the aggregation of platelets in response to ristocetin — ristocetin cofactor. This activity is usually reduced or absent in von Willebrand's syndrome, but is normal in haemophilia and has therefore been named by some as 'von Willebrand's factor' (VIIIR-Wf).

3 In patients with von Willebrand's syndrome, infusion of factor VIII causes a delayed and prolonged increase of factor VIII procoagulant activity which is thought to be due to either release or synthesis of factor VIII.

MAJOR ANTIGENIC SITES

1 Sites which react with heterologous antibodies to factor VIII. This reaction permits measurement of the concentration of factor VIII and this immunologic property is called factor VIII related antigen (VIIIR-ag).

Heterologous antibodies usually inhibit ristocetin cofactor, but may not inhibit procoagulant activity.

2 Sites which react with spontaneously occurring human antibodies to factor VIII. These antibodies inhibit factor VIII procoagulant activity, but do not inhibit ristocetin cofactor or interfere with the measurement of VIIIR-ag. These sites have been called factor VIII coagulant antigen (VIIIC-ag).

Factor VIII has a half life in the circulation of 8–12 hours, except in patients with von Willebrand's syndrome as explained above.

Diagnosis of carriers

It is possible to diagnose carriers of haemophilia by measurement of the ratio of factor VIII procoagulant activity and VIIIR-ag. This ratio is below the lowest normal value in 70–80% of obligatory carriers of haemophilia. By classical discriminant analysis and by incorporating the genetic probability of carrier status, it is possible to construct a computer programme which will predict the probability of carrier status based on the levels of factor VIII procoagulant activity and antigen. This is a major aid to genetic counselling, which should be offered to all members of the haemophiliac's family, but is of particular importance to maternal aunts and the sisters of the haemophiliac. The management of a patient with haemophilia is incomplete unless genetic counselling has been offered to all members of the family.

Prenatal diagnosis

Recently, evidence is accumulating that it may be possible to establish the diagnosis of haemophilia in male fetuses between 18–22 weeks of pregnancy. In this procedure, fetal blood is obtained by fetoscopy (for details of procedure see Chapter 21). Radioimmunoassays are used to measure VIIIC-ag and VIIIR-ag. After allowing for dilution of the fetal blood by contamination with amniotic fluid, a ratio of VIIIC-ag to VIIIR-ag can be calculated. In haemophiliacs, the VIIIC-ag has either been completely absent or below three per cent. The VIIIR-ag has been normal. In fetuses which are normal, the VIIIC-ag has been as low as 13%, but there has also been some reduction in VIIIR-ag. Much more investigation will be required before accurate criteria for diagnosis will be established.

Treatment

The bases of treatment are: (1) replacement of factor VIII, (2) restoration of normal function, (3) inhibition of fibrinolysis and (4) control of pain and prevention of drug addiction.

1 REPLACEMENT OF FACTOR VIII

The majority of spontaneous joint or soft tissue haemorrhages can be controlled by maintaining factor VIII levels above 15%. In the great majority of spontaneous bleeding episodes, a single factor VIII infusion to a level of 50% of normal will achieve haemostasis and maintain factor VIII levels above 15% for 24 hours.

There are some reports that in patients on home therapy, infusions of factor VIII to levels calculated to increase factor VIII to 10–20% may be sufficient to control bleeding episodes. While this may prove to be correct when the bleeding episode is treated almost immediately after its onset, it cannot yet be recommended for the treatment of patients usually seen in hospital.

The choice of product for replacement depends on its availability. High purity factor VIII concentrates have the major advantages of high concentration of factor VIII (low volume per injection) with low concentrations of other proteins, particularly fibrinogen and an accurately estimated dose of factor VIII units per bottle. Intermediate purity factor VIII concentrates or freeze dried cryoprecipitate are superior to 'wet' cryoprecipitate because these products can also be standardized to a known number of factor VIII units/ bottle and are more concentrated.

Estimation of dose The dose of factor VIII can be calculated by estimating the patient's plasma volume and using the definition that 'one factor VIII unit is that amount present in 1 ml of normal plasma'.

Thus, in a 30 kg child with a packed cell volume of 40%, the blood volume is 80 ml × 30, i.e. 2400 ml, and the plasma volume is 60% of the blood volume, i.e. 1400 ml. According to the definition of a unit of factor VIII, this patient will normally have 1400 units of factor VIII. To replace factor VIII to 50% of the normal level, 700 units of factor VIII will have to be infused. An alternative method of calculation is related to calculation of the increase in factor VIII activity in large groups of patients infused with a known amount of units of factor VIII. From these studies, it can be assumed that 1 unit of factor VIII/kg increases the factor VIII activity by two per cent. The number of factor VIII infusions required to control the most common types of bleeding and allow resumption of normal activity depends on the severity of bleeding and has been determined on empirical grounds. This is summarized in Table 3.1.

Table 3.1 The number of factor VIII infusions required to control the most common types of bleeding.

Types of bleeding	Number of infusions
Haemarthroses	1–3
Muscle and soft tissue	1–2
Bleeding threatening nerve compression, e.g. hip and forearm	3–6
Retroperitoneal haemorrhage	3–6
Intracranial	7–14
Oropharynx	3–6

Home treatment Families of children with haemophilia and the child himself may be taught to administer factor VIII concentrates at home. This reduces the patient's reliance on a hospital, encourages independence and greater freedom of movement. It was hoped that early treatment of joint haemorrhages may diminish their long term consequences. At present, there is no evidence that this has occurred. Nevertheless, home treatment is a well accepted and tried means of treatment in severe haemophiliacs and should be encouraged in children who require at least weekly infusions of factor VIII and are cooperative when they have an intravenous injection.

2 RESTORATION OF NORMAL FUNCTION

This is achieved by commencing physiotherapy as soon as pain has subsided. Immobilization of the joint in a splint may be required to control pain, but should be discontinued in 24–48 hours to permit joint mobilization. Initially, static exercises should be used, but active exercises and weight bearing should be actively encouraged within the limits of the patient's tolerance. In some patients with chronic joint deformity, physiotherapy may result in repeated haemorrhages and is best performed under cover of factor VIII infusions. Restoration of reasonable joint alignment may require prolonged traction. There is no place for forceful manipulation of deformed joints under anaesthesia and factor VIII cover.

3 INHIBITION OF FIBRINOLYSIS

This is of proven value in haemorrhages from the mouth and nose and may reduce bleeding after surgery. It should be avoided in renal bleeding as it may give rise to clot retention. Two agents are most commonly used: (1) epsilon aminocaproic acid 400 mg/kg in 6 hourly divided doses for 7–14 days (usual doses 8–16 gm/day); (2) tranexamic acid 2–4 g/day in 6 hourly divided doses.

Side-effects of antifibrinolytic drugs are unusual. Nausea and vomiting and an occasional skin rash may occur.

4 CONTROL OF PAIN AND PREVENTION OF DRUG ADDICTION

Bleeding into joints or muscles is often acutely painful. Prompt infusion of factor VIII and temporary immoblization in a non-circumferential splint will secure haemostasis and diminish pain. Prompt aspiration of swollen and painful joints under cover of factor VIII will immediately stop pain. It is possible, but unproven, that joint aspiration may decrease the rate of degenerative joint changes. When analgesics stronger then paracetamol have to be used, it has been the author's experience that, in children, rectal proladone (oxyiodone pectinate) has been effective and non-addictive, possibly because of the route of administration. The use of strongly addictive drugs administered orally or intravenously should be strictly avoided — these include morphine, dextromonamide and pentazocine.

TREATMENT OF HAEMOPHILIACS WITH SPONTANEOUSLY OCCURRING ANTIBODIES TO FACTOR VIII

Antibodies to factor VIII appear in 8–15% of severe haemophiliacs, usually before the age of 20 years. Half of the patients with antibodies to factor VIII have low levels of antibodies and do not have a major anamnestic response after infusion of factor VIII. These patients have been called 'low responders'. They appear to derive therapeutic benefit from standard or double doses of factor VIII concentrates. They also respond to infusions of prothrombin complex concentrates which possess general, but at present ill-defined, procoagulant activities. Usually, the prothrombin concentrates are effective when infused to 50% of plasma factor IX level. The effectiveness of the prothrombin complex concentrate should be demonstrated by a shortening of the non-activated PTT in *in vitro* tests and a shortening of the activated PTT in the patient within 2 hours of infusion of the concentrate. There is clear evidence that not all prothrombin complex concentrates are equally effective and the manufacturers' information on the effectiveness of their product should be sought prior to its use.

The other half of the patients have high or intermediate levels of antibody to factor VIII and respond with an anamnestic response to factor VIII infusion. Despite a failure to note an increase in factor VIII after its infusion, these patients may also sustain a haemostatic effect with standard or double doses of factor VIII. They also respond to infusions of prothrombin complex concentrates usually without an anamnestic response. Prothrombin complex concentrates are very useful in the treatment of these patients in that they are clinically effective for the majority of bleeds and allow a diminution of the antibody level to occur over a period of time. This gives the patient an opportunity to have effective treatment with factor VIII concentrates in case of severe haemorrhage that fails to respond adequately to prothrombin complex concentrates. In the case of life-threatening haemorrhages, bovine or porcine factor VIII may secure haemostatsis but antibodies to these products develop between 7–21 days. Plasmaphoresis and immunosuppression may be of value when all other resources have failed.

Elective surgery in haemophilia

Before undertaking elective surgery, the presence of antibodies to factor VIII should be excluded by specific tests rather than screening methods. Enquiries must be made to ascertain that there are sufficient stores of factor VIII for replacement. In children, synovectomy may be considered as an elective measure to diminish the frequency and severity of joint haemorrhages. There is some evidence that synovectomy may diminish the frequency and severity of joint bleeds temporarily. Synovectomy may result in a diminished range of movement and it is possible that the synovial membrane may regrow. For these reasons, it may be best to reserve this operation for children with frequent and painful joint bleeds who do not show bony cyst formation or subarticular cartilage erosion.

The most frequent operations in children are dental extractions and tonsillectomy. In the case of tonsillectomy or similar surgery, it is wise to determine the patient's response to factor VIII replacement before the operation, to ascertain the increase in factor VIII level per unit of factor VIII per kg and the factor VIII half life. For surgery, the factor VIII level should be maintained at a postinfusion value near 100% and a pre-infusion value of 50% for the first 4–5 days. Subsequently, the levels may be allowed to fall to a postinfusion value of 50% and a pre-infusion value of 25% for the next 3–5 days. Antibiotics should be administered promptly if there is any suspicion of infection.

Dental extraction

Antifibrinolytic therapy should be commenced 24 hours before extraction. Just before extraction, factor VIII should be given as a single dose to an estimated level of 50%. In cases associated with infection, postoperative antibiotics may reduce the incidence of secondary haemorrhage. Antifibrinolytic therapy should be continued for 10–14 days. More than one infusion of factor VIII is seldom required, but the patients should be reviewed 6–7 days postoperatively to ensure that there is no secondary haemorrhage. Special dental splinting is not required with this treatment regimen.

Psycho-social aspects of treatment

Haemophilia is a disease which involves the whole family. In the treatment of the child, it is desirable to mobilize all the family as active participants in the child's management. It is important to encourage the family to regard the haemophiliac as a family member with a disability, but not a disease. At all time, the management of bleeding episodes should be considered in conjunction with both the child and the family's future expectations. It is better for the child to experiment with activities that may result in a haemorrhage, rather than empirically forbid activities that the child may desire. Contact sports, bicycle riding and adventurous climbing can be dangerous, but their prohibition may cause more severe psychological disability than the treatment of haemorrhages induced by these activities. Most children will voluntarily abandon activities which precipitate haemorrhages.

Voluntary organizations of haemophiliacs, families and friends have played a major role in the education of haemophiliacs and the community into the special needs of haemophiliacs. Such organizations should be actively encouraged to take an interest in the hospital treatment facilities. Self help by the families is often of greater value and more cost effective than professional help.

The following are some aspects of environmental manipulation which are particularly helpful:

1 Living quarters should be on the ground floor.
2 There should be readily available telephone contact with the hospital department treating haemophilia.
3 An education programme for teachers who have 'bleeders' in their classes should be established and conducted by a medical officer.
4 A visiting community nurse may be able to alleviate medical and social problems and save trips to hospital.
5 A 'beeper' system will allow the parents of young children mobility and yet allow them to maintain contact with baby-sitters, other family members or school teachers.

CHRISTMAS DISEASE

This is inherited as a sex-linked recessive disorder with an incidence of 0.5–1/100 000 of population. The presenting clinical features and laboratory diagnosis have been described in Chapter 2.

Types and diagnosis of carriers

In the majority of patients, there is a parallel reduction of factor IX coagulant activity and antigen. The carriers of this type of Christmas disease also show reduction of coagulant and antigen levels to approximately 20–60% of normal. In a small proportion of patients, there is a slight but significant excess of factor IX antigen over coagulant activity. The carriers for this type of Christmas disease often show a more marked excess of antigen over coagulant activity. In a third group of patients, there is a marked excess of factor IX antigen and these patients often have a prolonged prothrombin time when measured with bovine thromboplastin. The carriers for this type of Christmas disease also show an excess of antigen.

Treatment

The principles of treatment are identical to haemophilia. Calculation of dose — only approximately 60–70% of the expected rise of factor IX is observed after its infusion. The dose should be calculated as in haemophilia and increased by one third. Alternatively, it can be assumed that 1 unit of factor IX/kg will increase factor IX by 1.3%

Factor IX has a half-life of approximately 24 hours and infusions need not be repeated any more frequently.

CHOICE OF PRODUCT FOR INFUSION

Prothrombin complex concentrates are a convenient and easy way to administer factor IX. Occasional thromboses have been observed following the use of prothrombin complex concentrates before adequate quality checks on the thrombogenic properties of the concentrates were employed. With these checks, thrombosis is a rare complication. There is suggestive, but as yet inconclusive, evidence that infusion of factor IX concentrates at weekly or 2 weekly intervals may prevent spontaneous haemorrhages.

VON WILLEBRAND'S SYNDROME

The term von Willebrand's syndrome is preferred over von Willebrand's disease because of the great variety of clinical presentations and laboratory investigations which occur in this disorder. The classical description of von Willebrand's disease was: (1) autosomal dominant inheritance, (2) prolonged bleeding time, (3) reduced factor VIII procoagulant activity and (4) reduced platelet adhesion by one or other *in vitro* test.

Since the introduction of more detailed investigations of the functional and immunological properties of factor VIII (see p. 16), it has become clear that the most sensitive laboratory investigation is the measurement of ristocetin cofactor as this, of all tests, is most often reduced or absent in von Willebrand's syndrome. Unlike haemophilia, the factor VIII related antigen is also frequently reduced in von Willebrand's syndrome and the reduction may parallel the reduction of ristocetin cofactor or, less frequently, that of procoagulant activity. In a small but clinically significant proportion of patients, it has been found that there is abnormal electrophoretic mobility of the factor VIII related antigen and that this may be associated with carbohydrate abnormalities of the factor VIII glycoprotein. These patients may have normal or near normal factor VIII procoagulant and antigen levels, but they have prolonged bleeding time and low ristocetin cofactor. Finally, patients have been reported with abnormal ristocetin cofactor and associated platelet function abnormalities.

In doubtful cases, investigations should be repeated on at least three occasions, at it has been shown that in some individuals with von Willebrand's disease factor VIII functional and antigenic activities can fluctuate widely. While all authorities agree that it is too early to propose a definite classification of the von Willebrand's syndrome, the following main types are well recognized and their laboratory findings are summarized in Table 3.2.

Table 3.2 Provisional classification of von Willebrand's syndrome (ETRO working party on vWd).

	Bleeding time	VIIIC	VIIIR-ag	VIIIR-Wf
Type I	Prolonged	Reduced	Reduced	Reduced
Type II	Prolonged	Normal or reduced	Normal or near normal	Reduced
Type III	Prolonged	Normal	Reduced	Reduced (normal)
Type IV	Normal Slightly prolonged	Reduced	Reduced	Reduced

Incidence

There is no accurate data on the incidence of von Willebrand's syndrome as defined by modern criteria. In the author's experience, it is the commonest congenital bleeding disorder, but is usually mild and not clinically significant unless the patient has suffered trauma or surgery. Patients with von Willebrand's disease and spontaneous bleeding are seen approximately half as often as those with haemophilia.

Genetic counselling

Genetic counselling is based on a 50% chance of occurrence in an autosomal dominant disorder. In rare instances, apparent haemostatically normal parents may have children with severe von Willebrand's disease. Investigation of such parents shows minor abnormalities on laboratory testing and it can be assumed that the children have homozygous disease with severe bleeding manifestations. Recently, prenatal diagnosis of homozygous von Willebrand's syndrome has been reported by showing severely reduced VIIIR-ag and VIIIC-ag in blood obtained by fetoscopy.

Treatment

The principles of treatment are similar to those of haemophilia. Infusion of factor VIII results in a delayed and prolonged increase in procoagulant activity, but the prolonged bleeding time and abnormal ristocetin cofactor are corrected for only approximately 2–4 hours. To control bleeding in von Willebrand's syndrome, factor VIII should be infused to a level of 50% and repeated, if required, at 24–48 hour intervals. If a single infusion of factor VIII does not stop the haemorrhage, the infusion should be repeated as factor VIII concentrates contain variable quantities of 'von Willebrand factor'. In general, cryoprecipitate has more 'von Willebrand factor' than intermediate or high purity preparations.

CONGENITAL PLATELET FUNCTION DISORDERS

Incidence

No reliable information is available. Clinical impressions suggest that they are less common than von Willebrand's syndrome and more common than Christmas disease. The most common cause of abnormalities of platelet function is ingestion of aspirin and this must be excluded with certainty before accepting the diagnosis of a congenital platelet function abnormality.

Inheritance

See Table 2.1.

Table 3.3 Classification of disorders of platelet function.

Site of major abnormality	Disease
Membrane	
Glycoprotein	Glanzmann's disease
Glycoprotein	Bernard-Soulier syndrome
Prostaglandin synthesis	'Aspirin-like' syndrome
Storage pool deficiency	Hermansky-Pudlak syndrome
	Wiscott-Aldrich syndrome
	Cheidak-Higashi syndrome
	Idiopathic
Deficient nucleotide metabolism	Glycogen storage disease Type 1
	Fructose 1–6 diphosphatase deficiency

Classification

A general classification and an approach to the diagnosis of congenital platelet disorders was outlined in Chapter 2. A more detailed classification is presented in Table 3.3.

Treatment

Patients and their families should be instructed to avoid aspirin, which can seriously aggravate bleeding episodes. Menorrhagia can often be diminished in severity by the use of oral contraceptive agents containing high concentrations of oestrogens. This form of treatment should only be undertaken if severe menorrhagia is present. In patients who require surgery, postoperative platelet transfusion may be required. If at all possible, this should be from a single HLA compatible donor.

RECOMMENDED READING

Haemophilia

BIGGS R. (1977) Haemophilia treatment in the UK from 1969–1974. *British Journal of Haematology* **35**, 487.

BIGGS R. (1978) *The Treatment of Haemophilia A and B and von Willebrand's Disease.* Blackwell Scientific Publications, Oxford.

BLOOM A.L. & PEAKE I.R. (1977) Factor VIII and its inherited disorders. *British Medical Bulletin* **33**, 219.

BLOOM A.L. (1978) Clotting factor concentrates for resistant haemophilia. *British Journal of Haematology* **40**, 21.

DUTHIE R.B., MATHEWS J.M., RIZZA C.R., STEEL W.M. & WOODS C.G. (1973) *The Management of Musculo-skeletal Problems in the Haemophilias.* Blackwell Scientific Publications, Oxford.

LUSHER J.M., SHAPIRO S.S., PALASCAK J.E., VIJAYA RAO A., LEVIVE P.H., BLATT P.M. & HAEMOPHILIA STUDY GROUP. (1980) Efficacy of prothrombin-complex concentrates in haemophiliacs with antibodies of factor VIII. *New England Journal of Medicine* **303**, 421.

RATNOFF O.D. & JONES P.K. (1977) The laboratory diagnosis of the carrier state for classic haemophilia. *Annals of Internal Medicine* **86**, 521.

Christmas disease

PAREKH U.R., MANNUCI M. & RUGGERI Z.M. (1978) Immunological heterogeneity of haemophilia B: a multicentre study of 98 kindreds. *British Journal of Haematology* **40**, 643.

Von Willebrand's syndrome

ITALIAN WORKING GROUP (1977) Spectrum of von Willebrand's disease: a study of 100 cases. *British Journal of Haematology* **35**, 101.

WEISS H.J. (1968) Von Willebrand's disease — diagnostic criteria. *Blood* **32**, 668.

Congenital platelet function disorders

HARDISTY R.M. (1977) Disorders of platelet function. *British Medical Bulletin* **33**, 207.

Chapter 4
Acquired Disorders of Haemostasis

DEVELOPMENT OF HAEMOSTASIS IN THE NEWBORN

Clotting factors do not pass the placental barrier, but are synthesized in the fetus. Platelets and megakaryocytes appear in the fetus by 11 weeks gestational age. Fibrinogen, the fibrinolytic mechanism and the prothrombin complex appear by 11–15 weeks of gestational age. In premature infants, the platelet count is normal, but platelet function studies suggest impairment of the platelet release reaction. Fibrinogen and factor VIII are usually normal, but the other coagulation factors are diminished. In the majority of reported studies, there have been levels of 30–60% of normal. Heparin does not cross the placental barrier, but oral anticoagulants do. Warfarin therapy during the first trimester has been associated with a high frequency of serious structural abnormalities in the fetus apparently due to its teratogenic effects. If maternal anticoagulation is required, it is recommended that heparin be used either throughout the pregnancy or in the first trimester and 2–3 weeks before term, so as to avoid the teratogenic and anticoagulant effects on the infant.

The most common acquired disorders of haemostasis are: (1) haemorrhagic disease of the newborn, (2) disseminated intravascular coagulation, (3) disorders of haemostasis associated with congenital heart disease, (4) disorders of haemostasis associated with renal disease and (5) drug-induced disorders of haemostasis.

HAEMORRHAGIC DISEASE OF THE NEWBORN

The coagulation enzymes of the prothrombin complex, factors II, X, IX and VII, require vitamin K for biological activity during their synthesis. These serine proteases have been found to have a number of γ-carboxyglutamic acid residues which are required for their functional activity in haemostasis. The residues are formed by carboxylation of glutamic acid after the enzyme has been assembled on the microsomes of liver cells. The carboxylation of glutamic acid to γ-carboxyglutamic acid requires vitamin K. Prothrombin which does not possess γ-carboxyglutamic acid fails to bind Ca^{2+} which is required for it to bind to phospholipid during the process of conversion of prothrombin to thrombin (see Fig. 1.3).

Haemorrhagic disease of the newborn results from a failure to supply vitamin K for carboxylation of the glutamic acid residues of the prothrombin complex. In part, this is due to the delayed synthesis of vitamin K by the bacteria that colonize the infant's large bowel, but there is also a low dietary intake of vitamin K, particularly in breast-fed babies.

The haemorrhagic symptoms usually appear between the second and fourth days of life. Gastrointestinal bleeding, nose bleeds or the appearance of cephalohaematomas are the most frequent signs. This condition is now rare, as parental administration of 100 μg of vitamin K_1 to every newborn infant has become a routine. Large doses of vitamin K_1 should be avoided, as this may cause haemolysis. Established haemorrhagic disease of the newborn should be treated by transfusion of whole blood and vitamin K_1.

If bleeding continues after these measures, infusion of a prothrombin complex concentrate may be given.

In sick children with diarrhoea and poor diet, or children on prolonged broad spectrum antibiotic treatment, vitamin K deficiency may also develop and cause a secondary form of haemorrhagic disease. Alertness to this possibility and estimation of the prothrombin time may result in early diagnosis and treatment with vitamin K_1 before haemorrhage has occurred.

DISSEMINATED INTRAVASCULAR COAGULATION (DIC)

This condition may complicate many disease processes; may be transient or persistent; of no clinical importance; or cause the death of the patient. There is much confusion about its frequency, diagnosis and treatment. A description of the interrelationships that are involved in the clinical syndrome of DIC may clarify some of this confusion.

Pathogenesis

In most circumstances, DIC results from the activation of coagulation, resulting in the production of thrombin. When the activation of coagulation enzymes exceeds the ability of the naturally occurring inhibitors of activated coagulation factors (antithrombin III) to neutralize them, there is generation of thrombin and deposition of fibrin with consumption of procoagulants. If the rate of consumption exceeds the rate of their production, there is depletion of procoagulants, particularly those with a short half-life (factor V, VII). Activation of Hageman factor (XII) results in activation of prekallikrein to kallikrein and high molecular weight kininogen to kinin. This can cause vasodilatation, shock and endothelial cell damage. Activation of Hageman factor and tissue damage also results in activation of fibrinolysis. The fibrinolytic enzyme plasmin may lyse fibrin and fibrinogen to produce fibrin degradation products (FDP) which have anticoagulant activity. These reactions are summarized in diagrammatic form in Figs 4.1 and 4.2.

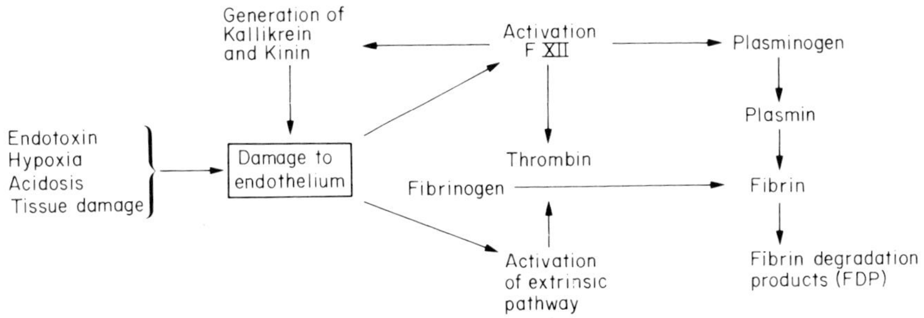

Fig. 4.1 Pathogenesis of DIC.

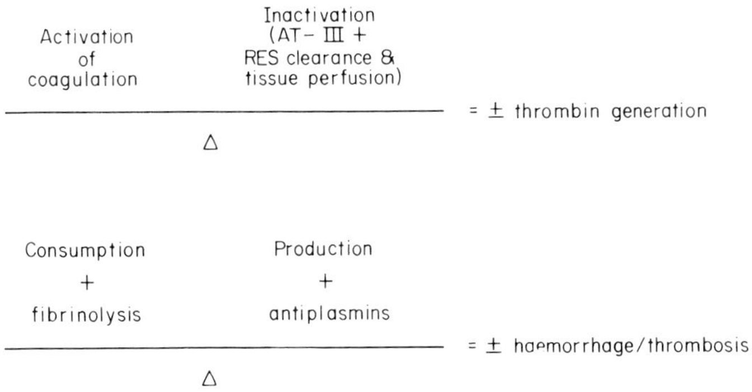

Fig. 4.2 Pathogenesis of DIC.

Diagnosis

In certain conditions, DIC is likely to complicate the course of the illness. An awareness of the association of DIC with these conditions may permit early diagnosis.

Conditions associated with DIC

INFECTIONS

1 *Bacterial* frequently, gram negative septicaemia, e.g. meningococcaemia, *Pseudomonas, Klebsiella, E. coli.* Occasionally, gram positive septicaemia, e.g. *Staphylococcus aureus*, streptococcal.
2 *Viral* viraemias, particularly herpes simplex in the newborn.
3 *Parastic* *Plasmodium falciparum* malaria, dengue fever.
4 *Fungal* septicaemias, e.g. *Candida.*
5 *Rickettsial* Rocky mountain spotted fever.

MALIGNANCY

In childhood acute promyelocytic leukaemia and, less often, myelomonocytic or myeloblastic leukaemia. There are only very occasional reports of DIC in acute lymphocytic leukaemia and disseminated neuroblastoma.

METABOLIC

Anoxia, acidosis, major tissue injury. This may complicate severe infections or respiratory distress in the newborn period.

MISCELLANEOUS

Purpura fulminans, snake bite, incompatible blood transfusion and heat stroke.

Clinical features

The major clinical features are bleeding from skin trauma sites, large ecchymoses and mucosal or renal bleeding. Shock and oliguria may be present and the children almost always look more sick than one may expect from the duration of the underlying disorders.

Laboratory diagnosis

Laboratory investigations are necessary to confirm the clinical diagnosis of DIC. The most commonly used show:

1 Prolongation of one stage prothrombin time.
2 Prolongation of activated or kaolin partial thromboplastin time.
3 The presence of fibrin monomers by protamine sulphate or ethanol gelation tests.
4 The presence of fibrin degradation products by immunological tests.
5 Thrombocytopenia.
6 Immunoassays show presence of fibrinopeptides A and B.

Treatment

The essential treatment is that for the underlying disorder. Shock, hypoxia and electrolyte disturbance should be treated by appropriate measures. If the patient has a self-limited illness for which there is specific therapy, e.g. septicaemia, no treatment for DIC may be required. In a minority of patients, correction of the haemostatic defects will be required if there is: (1) no specific treatment, (2) the treatment is unlikely to improve the underlying disorder rapidly and (3) the patient has severe bleeding manifestations.

This usually involves replacement of the coagulation factors that have been consumed and potentiation of inhibitors (AT-III) of the activated coagulation factors. This can be most readily achieved by infusing a prothrombin complex concentrate together with fresh frozen plasma (FFP), which is a source of AT-III, fibrinogen and intrinsic coagulation factor. Concentrates of AT-III may supersede the use of fresh frozen plasma. In order to potentiate the action of AT-III, heparin should be administered with the infusion of FFP. Usually, a loading dose of heparin of 200–400 units/kg is given followed by a constant infusion of 400–600 units/kg/24 hours. The higher loading dose of heparin is given to inactivate the thrombin activity which is present in patients with established DIC. The aim of this treatment is to correct towards normal values the prolonged PT and PTT, rather than to anticoagulate the patient. Heparin therapy can be discontinued when the underlying cause of DIC has been adequately controlled. If the underlying cause cannot be controlled, DIC usually responds poorly to treatment and the patient may die from haemorrhage. Antifibrinolytic agents have no role in the treatment of DIC.

There is no clinical evidence that heparin is useful in the treatment of suspected or established DIC in the newborn. In most neonatal clinics, suspected DIC is either treated by replacment of coagulation factors and AT-III or by exchange transfusion.

DISORDERS OF HAEMOSTASIS ASSOCIATED WITH CONGENITAL HEART DISEASE

Cyanotic congenital heart disease is associated with occasional thrombotic tendency in the first 1–2 years of life. More frequently, there is a haemorrhagic tendency which manifests itself as increased bleeding after surgery or trauma. Investigations of haemostasis in children with cyanosis and polycythaemia have shown that they have a prolonged one stage prothrombin time, low levels of factor II and VII and an 'aspirin like' defect of platelet function, as well as mild to moderate thrombocytopenia. All of these haemostatic defects occur more often in children with packed cell volume (PCV) greater than 60% and Hb greater than 16 g%. It is not known why these haemostatic defects occur. There is no evidence that they are caused by chronic low grade DIC. Infusion of prothrombin complex and platelet transfusion are often effective in treatment of postoperative bleeding in these children. In the author's experience, prophylactic infusions of these concentrates were effective in preventing bleeding in children requiring cardiac bypass surgery.

Occasionally, children with non-cyanotic congenital heart disease may have a haemostatic abnormality manifest by bleeding after surgery and a prolonged bleeding time in the presence of a normal platelet count. Platelet function studies are usually abnormal, showing either an 'aspirin like' defect or 'storage pool' disease.

DISORDERS OF HAEMOSTASIS ASSOCIATED WITH RENAL DISEASE

There has been much investigation on the role of the haemostatic mechanism in the pathogenesis of various types of renal disease. In humans, it is known that certain types of renal disease may be associated with haemostatic abnormalities.

In the nephrotic syndrome and some of the proliferative glomerulonephritis syndromes, there is a thrombotic tendency following endothelial damage, such as a femoral venepuncture. These patients often have elevated levels of procoagulants, hyperactive platelet aggregation and low AT-III levels. It is not known whether these haemostatic abnormalities are responsible for venous thrombosis after venepuncture, but deep vein punctures should be avoided in these children.

In the haemolytic uraemic syndrome (HUS), there is thrombocytopenia, shortened activated partial thromboplastin time, high levels of fibrinogen and procoagulants and raised FDP. Heparin and heparin plus streptokinase have been used in the treatment of these patients, and there is some evidence that these forms of treatment reduce the incidence of chronic renal damage following HUS. Whether or not these haemostatic abnormalities are causally related to HUS is still unclear and, at this stage, it is not possible to make definitive recommendations on the use of heparin and streptokinase in HUS. Recently, there is growing evidence that plasmaphoresis is effective in the treatment of thrombotic thrombocytopenic purpura (TTP). If TTP is an adult version of HUS, then plasmaphoresis may also prove successful in the treatment of HUS. Plasmaphoresis is used to eliminate antigen-antibody complexes which cause vascular damage. In uraemia, there may be bleeding associated with platelet function abnormalities. These can be corrected by haemodialysis.

DRUG INDUCED DISORDERS OF HAEMOSTASIS

There are many drugs that can affect platelet function *in vitro* and a smaller number that cause an alteration of platelet function *in vivo*. These are listed in Table 4.1. Only aspirin and high doses of penicillin related antibiotics have consistently been associated with a clinical bleeding tendency and platelet function abnormalities. Aspirin is therefore contraindicated in patients with congenital bleeding abnormalities and should be considered as a possible cause of an unexplained acquired bleeding tendency, particularly in children who present with gastrointestinal haemorrhage. The role of most of the drugs under investigation as antithrombotic agents in clinical medicine, is not yet established. Combinations of dipyridamole and aspirin or sulphinpyrazone, together with warfarin, are most frequently used as antithrombotic agents in the prevention of embolism following prosthetic cardiac valve replacement. Their role in this condition is not yet unequivocally established.

ANTICOAGULANT THERAPY

In childhood diseases, anticoagulant treatment is used infrequently because venous thrombosis is virtually never associated with fatal pulmonary embolism. Nevertheless, there are situations in which anticoagulant therapy is required to prevent the extension of a thrombus or the occurrence of arterial embolism.

Disorders associated with venous thrombosis in childhood

1 Nephrotic syndrome.
2 Prolonged intravenous catheterization.
3 Severe liver disease, including Reyes syndrome.
4 Severe dehydration with gastroenteritis.
5 Congenital antithrombin III deficiency.
6 Systemic lupus erythematosis with circulating anticoagulant and venous thrombosis.

Table 4.1 Drugs which inhibit platelet function.

Drug	Effect on platelet function and its mechanism	Some of clinical circumstances in which the drug is under investigation
Pyrimido-pyrimidine compounds, e.g. dipyridamole	Inhibition of platelet release reaction through inhibition of phosphodiesterase and an increase in cyclic AMP	In conjunction with other drugs. In cardiac valve prosthesis
Hydroxychloroquine	Inhibit aggregation and release reaction	Prevention of venous thrombosis
Non-steroidal anti-inflammatory drugs, e.g. aspirin, indomethacin, phenylbutazone and sulphinpyrazone	Inhibit platelet release reaction by inhibition of platelet cyclo-oxygenase. Weak inhibitors of thrombin induced aggregation	In conjunction with other drugs. Reduction of incidence of transient cerebral ischaemia (?) reduce incidence of venous thrombosis
Clorfibrate and Halofenate	Reduce sensitivity to release inducing agents	Myocardial ischaemia
Propranolol	Inhibition of second phase of ADP induced aggregation, diminished adherence to collagen	?
Penicillin and related antibiotics	Interfere with platelet release reaction	High doses cause bleeding tendency
Prostaglandin E_1, D_2 and Prostacyclin	Inhibit platelet release reaction	(?) feasibility of altering platelet reactions by modifying fatty acid composition of platelet membrane and synthesis of prostaglandins.

Disorders associated with arterial embolism

1 Heart valve replacement.
2 Arterial catheterization.

Treatment of venous thrombosis in childhood

It is necessary to elucidate the basic cause of the thrombosis. Haemostasis should be investigated to establish baseline levels for the PTT, PT and, if possible, a functional and immunological level of AT-III. Heparin is given intravenously at a bolus dose of 200 μ/kg followed by 400–600 μ/kg/24 hours in a continuous infusion. The aim of treatment is to prolong the PTT to 1½–2 times the normal value. If the underlying cause of the venous thrombosis is due to a readily reversible cause, e.g. intravenous catheterization or severe dehydration, prolonged anticoagulant treatment will not be required and heparin need not be continued for more than 10–14 days. If the cause of the thrombosis is not readily reversible, e.g. liver disease, nephrotic syndrome, then prolonged anticoagulation will be required. In such patients, treatment should consist of heparin and warfarin given simultaneously. Warfarin should be given in a loading dose of 7.5–20 mg during 48 hours followed by a maintenance dose of 2–8 mg/day. The effect of warfarin is monitored with the prothrombin time ratio, which should be between 1.5–3.0. A variety of tests can be used to monitor the effects of warfarin therapy. The thrombo test, using ox brain thromboplastin, is particularly sensitive to the presence of non-functional vitamin K dependant coagulation proteins, while prothrombin tests using human or rabbit brain thromboplastins are less sensitive. For monitoring, a lower index is acceptable for human and rabbit brain thromboplastins ($\simeq$ 1.5–2.2) than for ox brain thromboplastin (2.0–3.0).

Warfarin interacts with other drugs, which may increase its anticoagulant activity; these include chloral hydrate, aspirin, indomethacin. Full lists of drugs which can interact with warfarin are available from hospital pharmacies.

Treatment and prevention of arterial embolism

In patients with heart valve replacement, it may be necessary to prevent the risk of arterial embolization from valve thrombosis. The most frequently used regimens employ warfarin and inhibitors of platelet function. Dipyridamole 25–100 mg/day is the best documented antiplatelet agent but, recently, there has been much interest in the effects of aspirin and/or sulphinpyrazone.

THROMBOLYTIC THERAPY

Rarely, in children, it may be desirable to attempt thrombolytic therapy in case of life-threatening venous or arterial thrombosis. Such therapy may be used in an attempt to preserve a limb or restore circulation in the mesenteric or retinal vessels. It is contraindicated in the treatment of cerebral vascular thrombosis or embolism. If surgical embolectomy is not possible, these patients can be treated with streptokinase. Usually, it is not possible to determine the patients' resistance to streptokinase, as the agent is given under emergency circumstances. In children who are under 30 kg, a loading dose of 50 000–100 000 units followed by 5 000–10 000 units/hour for 48–72 hours, may be given. In children who are over 30 kg, the loading dose is between 100 000–250 000 units followed by a maintenance dose of 20 000–100 000/hour. Most recently, urokinase and plasminogen (glutamic acid containing form) have been used to achieve more effective clot lysis in adult patients.

RECOMMENDED READING

Haemostasis in newborn

Blezer W.A., Hakami N. & Shepard T.J. (1971) The development of hemostasis in the human fetus and newborn infant. *Journal of Pediatrics* **79**, 838.

Haemorrhagic disease of newborn

Abolli A.J. & Lamereas S. de (1962) Hemorrhagic disease of the newborn: Two forms with different hemostatic defects. *American Journal of Diseases of Childhood* **104**, 475.

Stenflo J. (1977) Vitamin K, prothrombin and γ-carboxyglutamic acid. *New England Journal of Medicine* **296**, 624.

DIC

Deykin D. (1970) The clinical challenge of disseminated intravascular coagulation. *New England Journal of Medicine* **283**, 636.

Ekert H. (1975) Disseminated intravascular coagulation in children. *Paediatrician* **4**, 227.

Seigal T., Seligsohn U., Aghai E. & Modan M. (1978) Clinical and laboratory aspects of disseminated intravascular coagulation (DIC): A study of 118 cases. *Thrombosis and Haemostasis* **39**, 122.

Congenital heart disease

Ekert H. & Dowling S.V. (1977) Platelet release abnormality and reduced prothrombin levels in children with cyanotic congenital heart disease. *Australian Paediatric Journal* **13**, 17.

Maurer H.M., McCue C.M., Caul J. & Still W.J.S. (1972) Impairment in platelet aggregation in congenital heart disease. *Blood* **40**, 207.

HUS

AVALOS J.S., VITACCO M., MOLINAS F., PENOLUER J. & GIANANTONIO C. (1970) Coagulation studies in the hemolytic-uremic syndrome. *Journal of Pediatrics* **74**, 538.

LIEBERMAN E. (1972) Hemolytic-uremic syndrome. *Journal of Pediatrics* **80**, 1.

MONNENS L., KLEYNEN F., MUNSTER P. VAN, SCHRETLEN E. & BONNERMAN A. (1972) Coagulation studies and streptokinase therapy in the haemolytic-uraemic syndrome. *Helvetica Paediatrica Acta* **27**, 45.

Drugs and platelets

PACKHAM M.A. & MUSTARD J.F. (1977) Clinical Pharmacology of platelets. *Blood* **50**, 555.

WEISS H.J. (1978) Anti-platelet therapy (part 1 of 2). *New England Journal of Medicine* **298**, 1344.

Anticoagulant therapy

BASU D., GALLUS A., HIRSH J. & CADE J. (1972) A prospective study of the value of monitoring heparin treatment with the activated partial thromboplastic time. *New England Journal of Medicine* **287**, 324.

HIRSH J., CADE J.F. & GALLUS A.S. (1972) Anticoagulants in pregnancy: A review of indications and complications. *American Heart Journal* **83**, 301.

WESSLER S. & GITEL S.N. (1979) Heparin: new concepts relevant to clinical use. *Blood* **53**, 525.

Thrombolytic therapy

FRATANTONI J.C., NESS P. & SIMON T.L. (1975) Thrombolytic therapy: Current status. *New England Journal of Medicine* **293**, 1073.

POWELL R.N. & EKERT H. (1974) Streptokinase, heparin and anti-platelet drugs in the hemolytic-uremic syndrome. *Journal of Pediatrics* **84**, 345.

Chapter 5
Thrombocytopenic Purpura

Thrombocytopenic purpura, either secondary to viral infection or idiopathic, is the most common of the platelet disorders. Other causes of thrombocytopenia are uncommon, but usually have a grave prognostic significance. They are listed at the end of this chapter. The pathogenesis, natural history and response to treatment of ITP will be described in detail.

Platelet production

Platelets are produced by multinucleated cells known as megakaryocytes which are predominantly situated in the bone marrow. Production of platelets is related to the megakaryocyte mass and the extent of DNA replication in the megakaryocyte. Megakaryocytes have from 2–32 n DNA content and the higher DNA content is associated with greater platelet production. There is good evidence that platelet production is regulated by a humoral substance called thrombopoietin which increases the number of megakaryocytes, intracellular mitoses and rate of platelet production.

IDIOPATHIC THROMBOCYTOPENIC PURPURA (ITP)

Clinical features

In childhood, the idiopathic connotation is often incorrect as thrombocytopenia frequently follows a well established viral infection, e.g. varicella, rubella, cyclomegalovirus, herpes simplex or EBV infection. Most often, there are coryzal symptoms two weeks before presentation; less often, there is a recent past history of varicella, rubella or measles. Occasionally, the development of the disorder may follow rubella or measles vaccination. In approximately one third of children, there is no history of predisposing causes and, in these children, there may be a subacute or chronic presentation.

The most common presenting factors are sudden onset of marked bruising on the extremities and trunk. There may be associated nose bleeding, gum bleeding, subconjunctival haemorrhages and, less often, gastrointestinal haemorrhage. The peak age incidence is between 2–8 years and girls are slightly more often affected than boys.

Examination of the patient confirms the widespread bruising and/or petechiae. In patients without an accompanying infection, the spleen is not palpable. In patients with active viral infections, there may be minor degrees of splenomegaly. Laboratory investigations show a low platelet count, which is often between 5–30 × 10^9/l. The haemoglobin is usually normal and the white cell count is normal or raised. Although the clinical presentation and blood examination are typical, the diagnosis should be confirmed by bone marrow aspiration. Bone marrow aspiration eliminates the possibility that the clinical presentation is due to leukaemia or aplastic anaemia. Most often, there are increased numbers of megakaryocytes with increased numbers of nuclei. Quantitation of megakaryocyte numbers has proven difficult. Less frequently, megakaryocyte number and morphology are normal. A reduction in the number of megakaryocytes in a technically satisfactory marrow aspirate is not compatible with the diagnosis of ITP.

Pathogenesis (Fig. 5.1)

Platelet survival is shortened markedly with a life span of less than 3 days compared with a normal of 8–10 days. The shortened life span is associated with a markedly increased rate of platelet turnover, indicating that ITP is due to an accelerated rate of platelet destruction. Recently, it has been shown that in chronic ITP the spleen produces large amounts of antibodies of the IgG class with platelet specificity. It has also been shown that platelets coated with these antibodies and a component of complement (C3) are readily phagocytosed by splenic macrophages.

It would thus appear that ITP is due to the production of antiplatelet antibodies and the phagocytosis of antibody coated platelets. The production of platelet antibodies in the spleen and the destruction of sensitized platelets

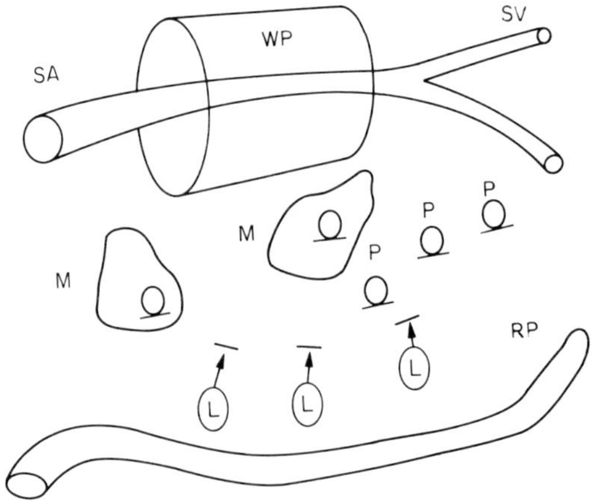

Fig. 5.1 Spleen involvement in ITP. (Modified from McMillan *et al* 1974.) SA: splenic artery; WP: white pulp; RP: red pulp; SV: splenic veins; L: lymphocytes producing IgG specific for platelets; P: platelets coated with IgG, M: splenic macrophages. Splenic lymphocytes produce IgG directed at platelets. Platelets coated with IgG are phagocytosed by splenic macrophages.

by splenic macrophages may explain why splenectomy cures ITP. Platelet destruction also occurs in other sites of the reticuloendothelial system, as the platelet lifespan may remain shortened after splenectomy and some patients with chronic ITP fail to respond to splenectomy.

Platelet survival studies may be used to demonstrate shortened platelet lifespan and to demonstrate major sites of platelet breakdown. This usually occurs in the spleen. High hepatic uptake of platelet radioactivity does not necessarily imply that uptake is not predominantly splenic during the second slower part of the survival curve which represents *in vivo* survival of platelets. In childhood ITP, it is unnecessary to measure platelet survival in order to make decisions on the need for, or response to, splenectomy.

Natural history and response to treatment

Acute onset with duration of symptoms of less than 2 weeks and age under 10 years are strongly associated with a self-limited course. Complete recovery occurs in 90% of these patients; in 75%, within 12 weeks, and in the remainder, within 26 weeks. In these patients, the platelet count has usually risen to over $20 \times 10^9/l$ at 3 weeks after presentation. Although steroids may accelerate the rise in the platelet count, there is no evidence that treatment with steroids increases the proportion of patients who achieve spontaneous remission. In 10% of children with an acute onset and short duration of symptoms, thrombocytopenia persists for longer than 26 weeks. These children can be considered to have chronic ITP. Permanent response to steroid therapy occurs in two thirds of these patients, but the remainder require splenectomy as thrombocytopenia recurs when steroids are stopped. Virtually all of these patients are cured by splenectomy.

Gradual onset with duration of symptoms for more than 2 weeks, often months or even years, and age greater than 10 years, are associated with only a 50% chance of spontaneous recovery. The platelet count at 3 weeks after presentation is a good indicator of prognosis; if it is $10 \times 10^9/l$ or less, spontaneous recovery is unlikely. In these patients, steroids may be commenced if the platelet count has shown no increase above the level at presentation after 6 weeks of observation, or if the platelet count has not risen above $20 \times 10^9/l$ after 12 weeks of observation. Permanent response to steroids occurs in only 20%. Response to splenectomy results in an elevation of the platelet count above $100 \times 10^9/l$ in 80–90%. In the remainder, thrombocytopenia persists, but even in these patients, the platelet count is increased to levels which are compatible with a normal lifestyle. This information is summarized in Fig. 5.2.

Treatment

A haemorrhagic tendency is most marked during the first week of the illness. In the majority of patients, strict rest in bed is all that is required to stop bruising and mucosal bleeding. The incidence of life-threatening haemor-

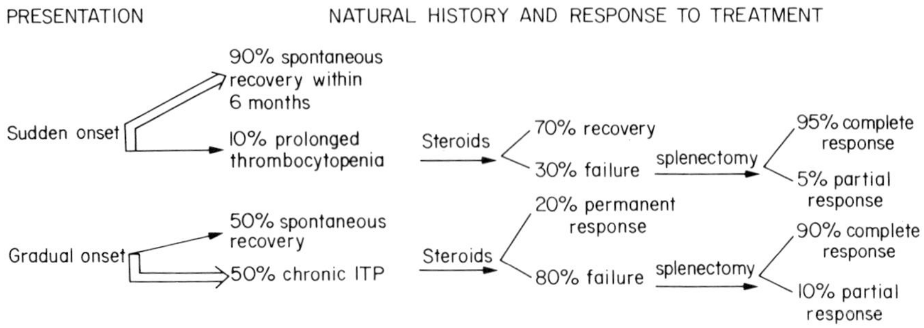

Fig. 5.2 The presentation, natural history and response to treatment.

rhages is very low. In two reviews of large numbers of patients, there were no fatalities in 229 children not treated with steroids, and two fatalities in 75 treated with steroids. As steroid treatment was only given to patients who, on clinical grounds, were judged to have severe haemorrhagic manifestations, it is not reasonable to conclude that steroids predispose to fatal haemorrhages. In the author's series, 80 children did not receive steroid therapy on admission during the years 1972–77. Of these children, only two were considered to require steroids and platelet transfusion for control of severe haemorrhagic manifestations and there were no deaths.

As steroid therapy is associated with unpleasant side-effects and the possibility of exacerbating viral infections, there appears to be no valid reason for its use in acute ITP. In the patients who have severe bleeding at presentation, e.g. gastronintestinal haemorrhage or profuse nose bleeding leading to anaemia, it is reasonable to administer prednisolone 2 mg/kg together with platelet transfusions. If this proves ineffective, then an emergency splenectomy may be required. In the author's experience, this has happened only once in 167 patients. In some patients, aspirin may have been given for treatment of a preceding infection 24–72 hours before the onset of bleeding. In such patients, bleeding will usually stop within 3–4 days as the proportion of normally functioning platelets increases to levels which prevent spontaneous haemorrhage.

When the acute phase of the illness has subsided, the patients may be observed at home, but activity should be restricted and the child should not return to school until there is recovery of the platelet counts to levels above 20×10^9/l and there are no haemorrhagic manifestations. Persistence of thrombocytopenia with a platelet count less than 10×10^9/l beyond an observation period of 3 weeks suggests that spontaneous recovery is unlikely. It is then reasonable to commence steroid therapy as outlined previously.

The usual course consists of prednisolone 2 mg/kg for 4 weeks followed by tapering of the dose for a further 2 weeks. Usually, there is an increase in the platelet count during the phase of steriod therapy, but in a significant proportion of patients, thrombocytopenia recurs when steriods are ceased (Fig. 5.2). If, after cessation of steroids, the platelet count falls to levels less than 20×10^9/l, then splenectomy will be required within days or weeks. If the platelet counts are above 20×10^9/l and there are no clinical haemorrhagic manifestations, it is reasonable to observe the patient for a total period of 6 months from presentation before recommending splenectomy, as in a small number, a spontaneous partial or complete recovery may occur during the observation period.

In childhood ITP, the response to splenectomy is excellent. A small number of children, however, continue to have persistent thrombocytopenia or recurrences of thrombocytopenia with infection. In these children, the platelet count is usually above $50 \times 10^9/l$ and they are able to pursue a normal life with only minor restrictions, such as avoiding contact sports.

There is good evidence that there is an increased risk of serious bacterial infections following splenectomy. These are most often due to pneumococcal and/or *Haemophilus influenzae* infections. In the absence of specific vaccines for these organisms, prophylactic antibiotic therapy using penicillin (Bicillin 200 000 u twice daily) appears reasonable, but with the advent of specific vaccines, prophylactic antibiotics may not be required. There is dispute on

Table 5.1 Secondary thrombocytopenia.

Condition	Associated findings
Thrombocytopenia absent radius (TAR)	Skeletal abnormalities absent radius
Aplastic anaemia	Marrow hypoplasia
Leukaemia	Marrow replacement
Disseminated neoplasma	Marrow infiltration
Viral infections	Hepatosplenomegaly
CMV	Positive viral studies
EBMV	
HSV	
Hepatic failure	Signs of liver disease
Haemolytic uremic syndrome	Renal disease
Polyarteritis and antigen-antibody complex disorders	Biopsy findings of arteritis antigen antibody complexes
Disseminated intravascular coagulation	Coagulation abnormalities
Drugs	History of drug exposure
Sulphomamides	
Quinine	
antineoplastic agents	
Chlorothiazide	
Phenylbutazone	
Chloramphenicol	
Penicillamine	
Methoin	
Troxidone	
Giant haemangioma	Haemangioma
Wiskott-Aldrich syndrome	Eczema, splenomegaly, failure to thrive
May-Hegglin anomaly	Giant platelets, leukocyte inclusion bodies
Post-transfusion purpura	Previous transfusion
Hypersplenism	Splenomegaly
Cyanotic congenital heart disease	Heart disease, polycythemia

the duration of prophylactic antibiotic therapy. Treatment should be continued for at least 2 years, but some claim that the risk of infections persist for a lifetime.

SECONDARY THROMBOCYTOPENIA

In addition to ITP, thrombocytopenia may also be found in association with the conditions listed in Table 5.1, most of which are self-explanatory and will not be further discussed. Only the drugs which most commonly cause thrombocytopenia are listed.

THROMBOCYTOPENIA IN THE NEWBORN PERIOD

Secondary to maternal ITP

This may occur whether the mother is thrombocytopenic or in remission. The infant is noted to have crops of petechiae at, or soon after, birth and they may be associated with bruising at sites of trauma, e.g. cephalohaematoma, bruised forceps marks. There is usually no hepatosplenomegaly. Spontaneous recovery occurs at between 3–6 weeks of life. In case of severe bleeding, it may be reasonable to perform exchange transfusion followed by platelet concentrate infusion. Such interference is only very rarely required.

Isoimmune purpura

Immunization may arise from fetomaternal passage of platelets. The diagnosis is suspected if there is no history of maternal ITP and the mother has a normal platelet count. The index of suspicion is heightened if successive pregnancies are involved. Methods for measurement of platelet antibodies are usually not good enough to detect maternal antibodies to platelets. Treatment is along similar lines to thrombocytopenia secondary to maternal ITP.

Maternal drug ingestion

Thromboctyopenia has been reported following maternal ingestion of quinine, thiazides and tolbutamide. The diagnosis can only be made by association and by excluding other causes. Treatment is as above.

Intrauterine infections

These can cause severe thrombocytopenia and should always be excluded before a diagnosis of some other cause of thrombocytopenia is made. The most common intrauterine infections associated with thrombocytopenia are rubella, disseminated herpes simplex, toxoplasmosis, cytomegalovirus, coxackie B and syphilis. Usually, the symptoms of thrombocytopenia are only one feature of a more generalized illness. Jaundice and hepatosplenomegaly are frequently found. Bone marrow findings are variable, and it is often reported that the number of megakaryocytes is reduced. The thrombocytopenia does not usually cause severe haemorrhagic manifestations, except in generalized herpes simplex infection where it appears to be associated with DIC and liver failure.

Other causes of thrombocytopenia in the newborn

KASABACH-MERRITT SYNDROME

The presence of a giant haemangioma is usually obvious, but if involves the liver or spleen it may not be immediately apparent. Usually, the thrombocytopenia is asymptomatic. If bleeding becomes a problem, the treatment is that of the giant haemangioma. Very occasionally, the haemangioma may be impossible to treat and there is a generalized haemorrhagic tendency. In this situation, it has been found that there is consumption of coagulation factors leading to DIC. Replacement of coagulation factors, together with careful heparin therapy, may reduce the bleeding tendency.

RENAL VEIN THROMBOSIS

Thrombocytopenia is a frequent accompanying feature of this illness, but there is no associated generalized bleeding tendency.

Thrombocytopenia in the newborn has also been described in abruptio placentae and a dead twin fetus.

RECOMMENDED READING

DIXON R.H. & ROSSE W.F. (1975) Platelet antibody in autoimmune thrombocytopenia. *British Journal of Haematology* **31**, 129.

LUSHER J.M. & ZEULZER W.W. (1966) Idiopathic thrombocytopenic purpura in childhood. *Journal of Pediatrics* **68**, 971.

MCMILLAN R., LONGMIRE R.L., YELENOSKY R., DONNELL R.L. & ARMSTRONG S. (1974) Quantitation of platelet-binding IgG produced *in vitro* by spleens from patients with idiopathic thrombocytopenic purpura. *New England Journal of Medicine* **291**, 812.

SIMONS S.M., MAIN C.A., YAISH H.M. & RUTZKY J. (1975) Idiopathic thrombocytopenic purpura in children. *Journal of Pediatrics* **87**, 16.

WILLIAMS N.B. & MAURER H.M. (1979) Acute idiopathic thrombocytopenic purpura in children. *American Journal of Hematology* **7**, 87.

Chapter 6
Neutropenia

At birth, there is frequently leukocytosis with counts as high as $40 \times 10^9/l$. These usually fall during the first week to an average of $20 \times 10^9/l$. Subsequently, the total white cell count ranges between $3–12 \times 10^9/l$. At birth, neutrophils predominate, but by one week of age, there is an increase in lymphocytes which predominate until there is again a predominance of neutrophils by the age of 8 years. The absolute neutrophil count beyond the newborn period ranges from $1.5–6.0 \times 10^9/l$. Neutropenia is defined as a neutrophil count below $1.5 \times 10^9/l$. In clinical practice, neutropenia presents most frequently in association with infection. It is necessary to establish whether the neutropenia is due to infection, marrow replacement, marrow toxicity or one of the congenital neutropenias. In most instances, a careful medical history, physical examination and a full blood examination will suffice to allow differentiation between marrow replacement and the other causes. The presence of marrow replacement can be confirmed by bone marrow aspiration. The differentiation between neutropenias due to infection, marrow toxicity and congenital neutropenias, is more difficult and will be discussed in this Chapter.

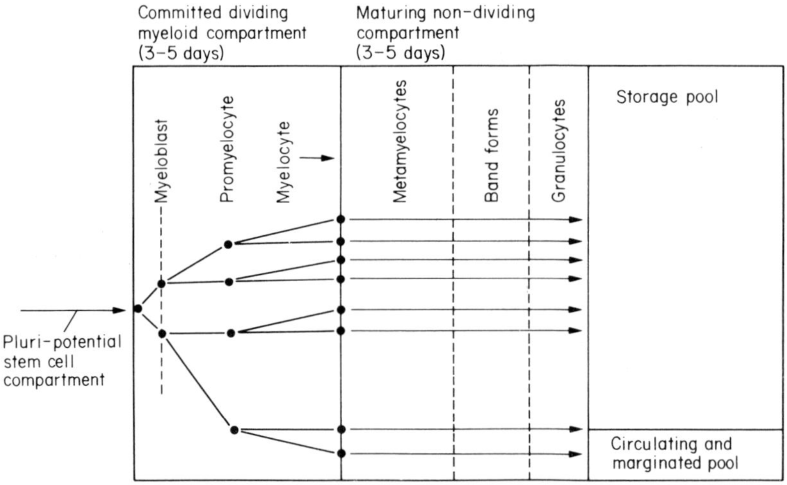

Fig. 6.1 Granulocyte differentiation and maturation.

PRODUCTION AND KINETICS OF GRANULOCYTES

Granulocytes are produced in the bone marrow and liberated into the blood stream where they undergo random destruction, with a mean half life of 7 hours. The production of granulocytes takes place by division and maturation of myeloid precursors. The earliest recognizable myeloid precursors are myeloblasts which divide and mature to promyelocytes and myelocytes in 3–5 days. These cells retain their potential for cell division. Further maturation of myelocytes gives rise to metamyelocytes, band cells and, finally, mature granulocytes, in 3–5 days. These cells are not capable of division. There is increasing evidence that the myeloid and erythroid series may share a common pluripotential stem cell which, under appropriate stimuli, may mature into a committed erythroid or granulocyte precursor. The production of granulocytes can be diagrammatically illustrated as shown in Fig. 6.1.

Methods of investigation

In clinical practice, neutropenia not due to leukaemia, marrow infiltration by malignant cells or aplastic anaemia is most often secondary to a chronic infection. Viral infections are most often associated with neutropenia which may last for some days or even weeks. The pathogenesis is shown in Fig. 6.2. The most useful clinical indication that neutropenia may be due to infection is the presence of failure to thrive, hepatosplenomegaly and lymphadenopathy. Investigations are:

1 Document presence of infections.
2 Diagnose infectious agent.
3 Observe blood counts for at least 3 weeks.

Frequently, the decision as to whether the neutropenia is primary or secondary to infection cannot be made without a period of observation of 3–6 weeks. During this time, blood examinations should be performed regularly to determine whether there is recovery and to exclude the presence of congenital neutropenia.

A less common but important and often readily distinguishable cause of neutropenia is marrow toxicity due to ingestion of certain drugs. The most important of these are co-trimoxazole, phenothiazone derivatives, tolbuta-

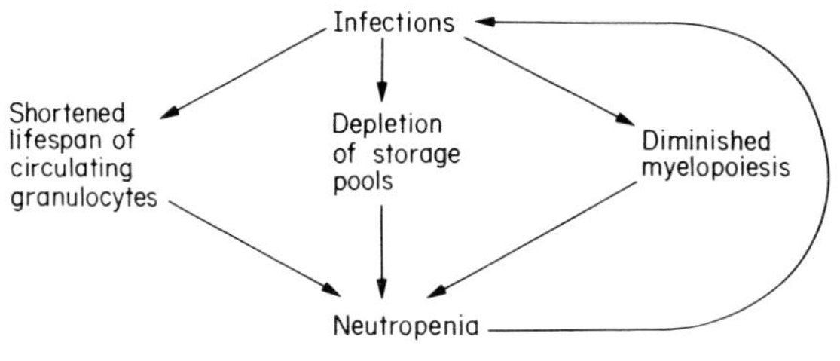

Fig. 6.2 Likely pathogenesis of neutropenia in chronic infections.

mide, chlorothiazide and antithyroid agents. A comprehensive list of drugs which have been reported to be associated with neutropenia, can be obtained from adverse drug reaction registers. The clinical diagnosis is made on the basis of history of drug exposure and by recovery of the neutrophil count 7–21 days after cessation of the responsible agent. Useful investigations are:

1 Document drug exposure and the date the last dose of drug was taken.

2 Confirm that the particular drug has previously been associated with neutropenia.

3 Observe blood counts for at least 3 weeks.

There are no adequate laboratory investigations to confirm that neutropenia has been caused by drug exposure. Marrow aspiration may show any one of the morphological features described below.

If at the end of a period of 3–6 weeks' observation the patient remains neutropenic, investigations for the aetiology of primary neutropenia should be undertaken. These centre on the following mechanisms: (1) failure of production, (2) excessive destruction, (3) failure to release from stores of marginated compartments and (4) failure to migrate to sites of infection.

Failure of production

Bone marrow aspiration gives some indication of the ability to produce myeloid precursors. In patients with a total or near total failure of myeloid production, there is a reversal of the normal myeloid-erythroid ratio and a paucity of all myeloid precursors. In the more common situations in which there is a partial failure of production, there may be a preponderance of early myeloid precursors with a lack of mature cells. This is due to exhaustion of the marrow storage granulocyte pool which reflects the diminished production of granulocytes. The only remaining myeloid cells in the marrow are those early precursors which do not enter the circulation. This marrow picture has been called 'maturation arrest', but does not, in fact, represent a true arrest of maturation beyond the myelocyte level. It is, however, possible that in some patients with neutropenia, there may be a true arrest of maturation. A normal marrow aspirate may also be seen in patients with reduced production if it happens that the marrow storage pools of granulocytes are only partially depleted and the patient is free of infection at the time of the marrow aspiration.

A rather special picture may occur in patients with partial failure of granulocyte production which gives rise to the clinical syndrome of cyclic neutropenia. If the bone marrow aspiration is performed before the nadir of the neutrophil count, there is 'maturation arrest'. The bone marrow picture returns to normal when the aspirate is performed at, or soon after, the nadir of the neutrophil count.

A new technique that may prove helpful in the investigation of failure of granulocyte production is bone marrow culture in soft agar or other suitable culture media. Under normal circumstances, culture of bone marrow produces 30–80 mixed colonies of granulocytes and macrophages per 10^5

nucleated cells plated. If there is a lack of normal granulocyte precursors, or if there are inhibitors to normal myeloid production, colony growth in soft agar may be impaired. To differentiate between reduced precursors and inhibitors to myeloid production, the marrow under investigation may be washed free of the inhibiting serum prior to culture and normal marrow may be cultured in the presence of the patient's inhibitor containing serum. Cell mediated inhibition of *committed* granulocyte precursors can be identified by mixing the test and a normal marrow and comparing the growth of colonies to that in either marrow, cultured in isolation under optimal conditions.

Excessive destruction

Hypersplenism is the most common cause of excessive granulocyte destruction, but this is usually clinically obvious because of the associated splenomegaly and other clinical and laboratory features of hypersplenism. Neutropenia may also occur with autoimmune diseases such as systemic lupus erythematosus, but is often an incidental finding rather than the cause of the patient's presentation. Excessive destruction of neutrophils may be confirmed by neutrophil turnover studies using DFP^{32} labelled granulocytes. The investigation is difficult to perform in children and is seldom used. Investigations for destruction of granulocytes in the marrow have been described above.

Failure to release stores

The marginated pool of granulocytes can be mobilized by infusion of 0.03 ml/kg of 1:10 000 adrenaline. The marginated pool is mobilized within 20 minutes of adrenaline administration. The marrow pool can be mobilized by infusion of 100 mg of hydrocortisone with hourly neutrophil counts for 6 hours. Although hydrocortisone may not be as good as etiocholanalone, it is better tolerated by the patients.

Failure to migrate to sites of infection

This may be tested by the Rebuck skin window technique.

The cause of neutropenia, not due to infection or drug exposure, the usual clinical diagnoses and the relevant investigations are shown in Table 6.1. These diseases are described in greater detail.

CONGENITAL NEUTROPENIAS

Cyclic

This disease appears to be due to partial failure of myeloid production.

Neutropenia occurs in cycles of approximately 3 weeks. The cyclic pattern may be altered by coincidental infection. Children with this disorder usually have frequent upper respiratory tract infections and often have gingivitis. Pneumonia may occasionally occur. Life-threatening infections are rare. The diagnosis is confirmed by the presence of the cyclical pattern of neutropenia with compensatory increase in monocytes at the nadir of the neutrophil count. In some children, the cyclical pattern is temporary and there may be complete recovery to normal counts. In the author's experience, this has

Table 6.1 Clinical diagnoses and investigations of neutropenia not due to infection or drug toxicity.

Cause of neutropenia	Usual clinical diagnosis	Relevant investigation
Failure of production	Cyclic neutropenia Chronic neutropenia	(1) Twice weekly FBE for 3 weeks (2) Bone marrow aspiration: reduced myeloid precursors 'maturation arrest' normal marrow (3) Bone marrow culture reduced colonies
Excessive destruction	Autoimmune Isoimmune Idiopathic	(1) Bone marrow aspiration: normal marrow or 'maturation arrest' (2) Bone marrow culture reduced colonies, improved by washing marrow. Bone marrow and/or serum inhibit(s) colony production of normal marrow (3) Reduced life span of DFP^{32} labelled granulocytes (4) Demonstrable white cell antibodies (5) Response to immunosuppressive therapy
Failure to release stores		(1) Normal or hypercellular marrow aspirate (2) Neutrophilia following adrenaline or hydrocortisone stimulation (3) Increased marrow store with DFP^{32} studies
Failure to migrate	Lazy leucocyte syndrome	(1) Normal or hypercellular marrow aspirate (2) Increased marrow stores with DFP^{32} (3) Negative Rebuck window (4) No response to hydrocortisone

occurred in children who have associated diminution of immunoglobulin levels and, in particular, IgG. Treatment with gammaglobulin has resulted in a diminished frequency of infections and this was followed by disappearance of cyclical neutropenia. In other children, cyclical neutropenia may progress to chronic neutropenia with a higher incidence of serious infections.

However, in the majority of children with cyclic neutropenia, the disease is life-long. There is no specific treatment, but the family has to be warned of the potentially serious nature of infections and early antibiotic treatment of established infections is required. There is no evidence that prophylactic antibiotics are of value. Cyclic neutropenia can occasionally be associated with exocrine pancreatic insufficiency.

Chronic

This disorder appears to be as frequent as cyclic neutropenia. At least three forms may be recognized.

1 Severe agranulocytosis presenting in early childhood. There is recessive inheritance and the condition is often fatal in early childhood. The disease was described as 'infantile genetic agranulocytocis' by Kostman in 1956.

2 Familial benign neutropenia which appears to have a dominant inheritance and patients with it may survive to adult life.

3 Chronic benign granulocytopenia which is the most common, shows no familial tendency and tends to improve with age.

Children with chronic neutropenia have frequent upper respiratory infections and often poor weight gain. Pneumonia, septicaemia and liver abscesses occur occasionally and may be life-threatening. The diagnosis is made on the basis of persistent neutropenia, usually without a compensatory monocytosis. Occasionally, there is an associated decrease in levels of IgG and cell mediated immunity. These children have a more severe clinical course and, if they do not die of infections, may develop malignant lymphoma in later childhood. Chronic neutropenia may also be associated with exocrine pancreatic insufficiency, growth retardation, metaphyseal dysostosis, anaemia, thrombocytopenia and galactosuria. This has been called the Schwachman syndrome.

The treatment of chronic neutropenia requires vigorous antibiotic treatment early in the course of infections. Infections which are more serious than gingivitis, tonsillitis or otitis media, should be treated with intravenous antibiotics after appropriate blood cultures have been taken. As some children with chronic neutropenia may show a spontaneous recovery and, in most, the tendency to frequent and severe infections diminishes with age, it is particularly important to maintain a watchful policy for severe infections during early childhood. This may be best achieved by regular follow-up in a specialized haematology unit.

IMMUNE NEUTROPENIA

Isoimmune

Isoimmune neutropenia is a rare cause of neutropenia at birth. The clinical clue to its presence is the occurrence of neutropenia in successive births. The condition can be confirmed by demonstration of antibodies in maternal blood to leucocytes of the same leucocyte type or those of the infant. Such tests can only be performed in specialized laboratories. The neutropenia may persist for up to 60 days, but eventually there is full recovery. Precautions against exposure to infection during the period of neutropenia may be life-saving.

Autoimmune

This may be due to a maternal autoimmune disorder or systematic lupus (SLE) in the child. Significant neutropenia with SLE is uncommon. Recently, a number of patients have been described with neutropenia occurring late in childhood or early adult life. These patients appear to have autoantibodies to neutrophils, but no other manifestations of an autoimmune disorder. In some patients, splenectomy has been followed by a recovery of the neutrophil count. Others have shown recovery following treatment with cyclophosphamide. Although this newly described condition is rare, it is important to remember that it may be present in children with late onset of neutropenia. The investigations required to document its presence are summarized in Table 6.1.

NEUTROPENIA IN HYPERSPLENISM

This is usually obvious and is associated with splenomegaly. Neutropenia is seldom severe and is usually associated with more profound anaemia than thrombocytopenia. It is very rarely necessary to perform splenectomy for the neutropenia.

LAZY LEUCOCYTE SYNDROME

This condition appears to be due to a failure of egress of neutrophils from the marrow. There are frequent upper respiratory tract infections. The diagnosis is confirmed by the tests outlined in Table 6.1.

Neutropenia has also been described in association with rare inborn errors of metabolism. These are idiopathic hyperglycenaemia, isovaleric acidaemia and methylmalonic acidaemia.

RECOMMENDED READING

BAEHNER R.L. (1974) Molecular basis for functional disorders of phagocytes. *Journal of Pediatrics* **84**, 317.

CLINE M.H. (1975) *The White Cell*, Chapters 2, 3, 8 & 9. Harvard University Press, Cambridge, Mass.

CLINE M.J., OPETZ G., SAXON A., FAHEY J.L. & GALDE D.W. (1976) Autoimmune panleukopenia. *New England Journal of Medicine* **295**, 1489.

KANDER E. & MAUER A.M. (1966) Neutropenias of childhood. *Journal of Pediatrics* **69**, 147.

SAUNDERS E.F., GALL G. & FREEDMAN M.H. (1979) Granulopoiesis in Schwachman's syndrome (pancreatic insufficiency and bone marrow dysfunction). *Pediatrics* **64**, 515.

SCHWACHMAN H., DIAMOND I.K., OSKI F.A. & KHAN KON-T. (1964) The syndrome of pancreatic insufficiency and bone marrow dysfunction. *Journal of Pediatrics* **65**, 645.

Chapter 7
The Leukaemias

Classification

In childhood, 85% of the leukaemias are acute lymphocytic, the remainder consisting of acute myeloblastic leukaemia and its various subgroups, chronic myeloid leukaemia of the adult and juvenile type and, very rarely, histiocytic or erythroblastic leukaemia (Table 7.1). Chronic lymphatic leukaemia is so rare in childhood that, for practical purposes, it may be said not to occur. Acute lymphocytic leukaemia will be described in some detail while, in the other leukaemias, only aspects of special paediatric interest will be discussed.

THEORETICAL BACKGROUND TO TREATMENT

At the time of diagnosis, it is estimated that the leukaemic cell load is about 10^{10}–10^{12} cells. A high proportion (60–90%) of these cells are capable of passing through the cell cycle (Fig. 7.1), but at any one time only a small number of cells are synthesizing DNA (Fig. 7.2). These cells are most susceptible to anti-cancer drugs, as the majority of these drugs act by interfering with DNA synthesis, organization or repair. The generation time of leukaemia cells is about 47–55 hours, while that of normal marrow and gut cells varies from 24–36 hours. When anti-cancer drugs are administered, both normal and leukaemic cells that are in the DNA synthetic phase (S) of the cell

Table 7.1 Types of childhood leukaemia.

Acute
Acute lymphocytic
Acute myeloblastic
Myelomonocytic
Promyelocytic
Monocytic
Erythroblastic
Histiocytic
Chronic
Chronic myeloid leukaemia adult type
Juvenile chronic myeloid leukaemia (myeloproliferative syndrome)

cycle will be killed or damaged. The proportion of normal-leukaemic cells killed will depend on the relative sensitivity of the cells to the drugs used, and the number of normal and leukaemic cells that are in the S phase during the time that there are pharmacological concentrations of the drugs. As leukaemic cells have a longer doubling time, it is possible that a significant number of leukaemic cells will be in the S phase during any given time that there are pharmacological drug concentrations. On the other hand, the shorter doubling time of normal cells means that more normal than leukaemic cells will be entering the S phase.

Whatever the ratio of normal:leukaemic cell kill there may be during drug treatment, when it is stopped, the short doubling time of normal cells usually ensures that they return to pretreatment levels before the leukaemic cells. If chemotherapy is repeated when the normal cells have recovered, a reduction of the leukaemic cells number relative to normal cells would have been

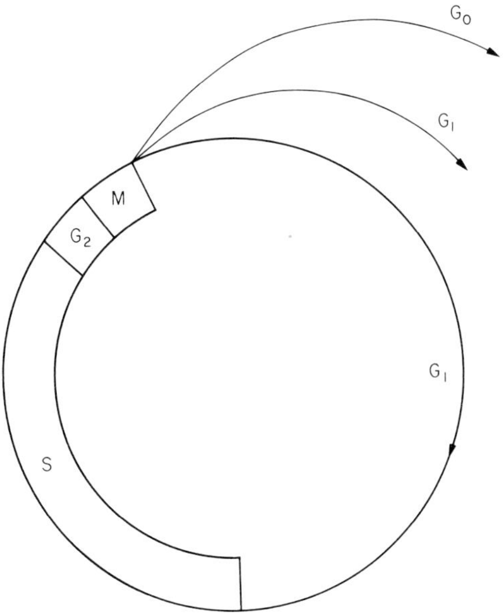

Fig. 7.1 Cell cycle. S: phase of DNA synthesis and organization; G_2: resting phase prior to mitosis; M: mitosis; G_1: resting phase associated with protein synthesis. Some cells remain in G_1 phase for prolonged periods of time, but can be recruited into cell cycle under certain circumstances such as depletion of the cycling pool, G_0: true resting cells which have permanently lost their proliferative potential.

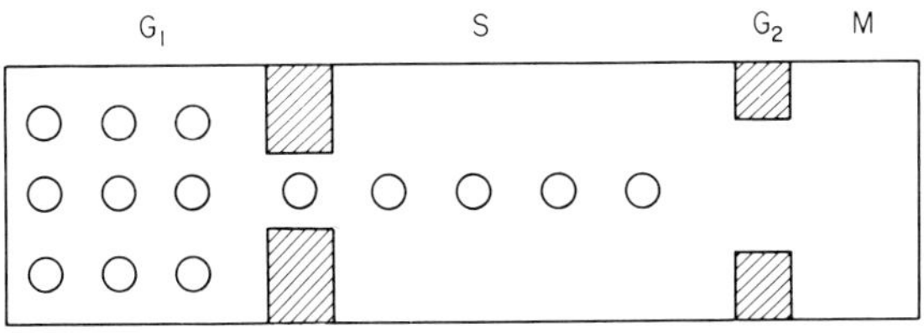

Fig. 7.2 Progress of cell through cell cycle. Tumor cells do not all simultaneously pass from G_1 to S. The number of cells in S phase at any one time is considerably less than in the G_1 phase.

achieved and, with repeated courses of chemotherapy, leukaemic cells can be eradicated without reducing normal cell numbers (Fig. 7.3).

It is generally considered that the doubling time of leukaemic cells is not affected by reducing their numbers. There is no direct evidence that this applies to human leukaemia. If in human leukaemia, there is a plateau of growth of both high and low cell numbers, then, after initial chemotherapy, a diminishing proportion of leukaemic cells will enter the S phase and cytotoxic therapy will result in a greater kill of normal than leukaemic cells. If this is the case, then the most effective leukaemic cell kill can be achieved with intensive chemotherapy during the induction phase of treatment.

There is evidence that tumour cells have, or can develop, increased levels of enzymes directed at DNA synthesis and repair. This may be one mechanism of drug resistance. Empirically, it has been confirmed that combinations of drugs are more effective in eradicating leukaemic cells and, therefore, presumably preventing the appearance of drug resistant cells. On these grounds, it is also preferable in situations of drug toxicity to postpone chemotherapy rather than reduce its dose, as dose reduction may allow induction of enzymes which can overcome the cytotoxic effects of the drugs.

It hase been amply confirmed that there are pharmacologic sanctuaries in leukaemia. In these sites, there is a barrier to the entry of cytotoxic drugs in effective concentrations. The major sanctuary is the CNS because of the blood-brain barrier. In order to effectively eradicate leukaemic cells from the CNS, it is necessary to administer effective therapy before there are signs and symptoms of CNS infiltration. Other known sanctuaries are the testes, iris and occasionally scalp skin when tourniquets are used to prevent hair loss due to chemotherapy.

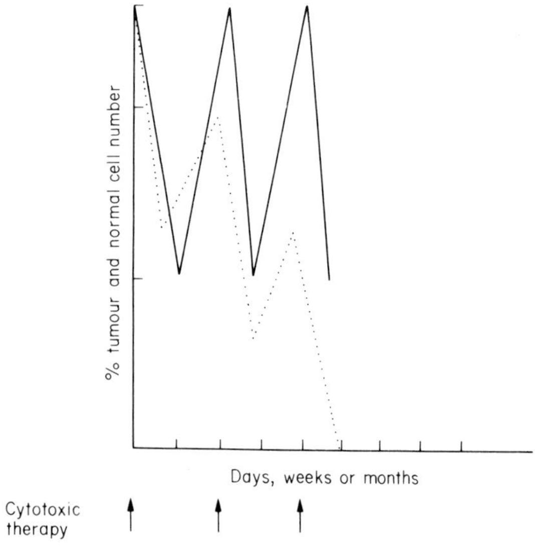

Fig. 7.3 Stepwise reduction of leukaemia cell number. Intermittent chemotherapy causes stepwise reduction of leukaemia cells without the destruction of normal cell population because of the long doubling time of leukaemic cells and their slower rate of recovery from the effects of cytotoxic therapy. Solid line: normal cells; dotted line: leukaemia cells.

ACUTE LYMPHOCYTIC LEUKAEMIA

Incidence and aetiology

Acute lymphocytic leukaemia is the commonest childhood malignancy. Its incidence is approximately 4 per 100 000 children under the age of 15. The risk of a child developing leukaemia has been caculated as 1:2880. Its peak incidence is between the ages of 2–5 years, and both sexes are equally affected. The cause of leukaemia remains unknown and, in general, it is rare to find a plausible predisposing cause. Rare predisposing factors are:

1 Chromosome abnormalities, particularly Down's syndrome, Bloom's syndrome, presence of the Philadelphia chromosome, chromosome translocation $14q^{+}8q^{-}$.

2 Exposure to known carcinogenic agents in the environment, e.g. radiation.

3 Immune deficiencies, e.g. ataxiatelangiectasia, Bruton's agammaglobulinaemia.

Large-scale surveys of families with leukaemia and cancer indicate that these families have double the incidence of cancer than in a control group of patients without malignancy. If one monozygotic twin develops leukaemia, there is a 20% chance that the other twin will also develop leukaemia within the next 6 months.

Clinical presentation

Most frequently, the patients present with the symptoms of anaemia and bone pain. Presentation with haemorrhagic symptoms is very rare. In childhood, bone pain may present as excessive tiredness, unexplained bouts of weeping, growing pains, refusal to attend school, or a limp. Occasionally, severe backache may be present. Fleeting bone and joint pain may lead to a diagnosis of rheumatic fever or rheumatoid arthritis. Pyrexia with or without an obvious source of infection is frequently present, but is not usually an initial presenting feature. Headaches, convulsions or the appearance of lumps, constitute other rare forms of presentation.

Examination of the patients usually confirms pallor and bruising. In 70% of patients, there is significant hepatosplenomegaly and lymphadenopathy. Superior mediastinal enlargement, with obstruction of venous return, occurs in less than 5% of patients. Fundal examination is usually normal and papilloedema at presentation occurs in less than 1% of patients.

Diagnosis

The diagnosis is established on the basis of the peripheral blood count and bone marrow aspiration. In 60% of patients, there is a low haemoglobin and platelet count, with a leucocytosis between 10–30 × 10^9/l. The differential count shows neutropenia and the presence of either abnormal lymphocyte-like cells or lymphoblasts. In 20% of patients, the leucocyte count exceeds 30×10^9/l and the differential count frequently shows only blasts. Males predominate in this group of patients and, surprisingly, the haemoglobin level is often well maintained. In another 20% of patients, the full blood examination shows anaemia, leucopenia and thrombocytopenia. The differential count shows a profound neutropenia and no peripheral blasts are present. This type of blood picture, when associated with leukaemic marrow infiltration, is sometimes labelled as 'aleukaemic leukaemia'.

A bone marrow aspiration is always necessary to definitely confirm the presence of leukaemia and define its morphological type. The bone marrow should also be used for definition of the surface markers on the blast cells and for chromosome analysis.

Morphology and cytochemistry

In acute lymphocytic leukaemia, the bone marrow is most often nearly completely replaced by lymphoblasts. These cells vary in size from approximately the size of a lymphocyte 2–4 times its size. There may be great variability of cell size. There is always a high nuclear-cytoplasmic ratio. The nucleus has none or few nucleoli and there is frequently some condensation of chromatin. Often, there is a perinuclear halo. The cytoplasm of the cells stains a light blue with Romanowsky stains and contains none or a few granules only.

Experienced haematologists can determine the type of leukaemia on morphological examination of the marrow aspirate in some 80% of patients. Confirmation of the diagnosis can be obtained by cytochemical stains. In ALL, the blasts are often PAS positive and Sudan black B negative. Terminal deoxynucleotidyl transferase (TdT) activity appears to be specific for ALL blasts. With the use of cytochemical stains, the great majority of patients can be classified into the acute lymphocytic or myeloblastic groups. Recently, some authorities have claimed that the size and maturity of the lymphoblasts correlate with the prognosis. This has given rise to the Franco-American-British (FAB) classification of L_1 L_2 L_3 lymphoblastic leukaemias. The morphologic details of each type is beyond the scope of this text. In general, in the L_1 type small blasts with homogenous nuclear chromatin predominate and the nucleoli are not visible or inconspicuous. In the L_2 type the blasts may be large but there is heterogeneity in size and nuclear chromatin and one or more nucleoli are present. In the L_3 type, the cells are large and homogenous, chromatin is stippled and homogenous and nucleoli are prominent. The L_1 type is said to have the best and the L_3 the worst prognosis.

Prognostic factors

It is well established that certain clinical and laboratory features at presentation may be used to approximately predict the likely response to treatment. There is no doubt that, with further investigation, a greater number of immunological and biochemical markers with prognostic value may be found. The following are the most important prognostic features:

1 *Age* Children under the age of 2 years and over the age of 12 years have a worse prognosis than children between that ages of 2–12 years. Children under the age of 12 months have a particularly poor prognosis.

2 *Sex* Girls over the age of 10 years with low white cells counts at diagnosis have a significantly greater long-term relapse rate than boys with the same presenting features. Boys with high white cell counts at diagnosis have a significantly higher relapse rate than girls with the same presenting features. In the remaining patients, it would appear that girls have a significantly better long-term prognosis.

3 *Organomegaly* In general, the larger the liver, spleen or lymph nodes, the poorer the prognosis. In particular, marked enlargement of the liver is a sign of poor prognosis.

4 *Mediastinal lymphadenopathy* The presence of a mediastinal mass is often considered to be a sign of poor prognosis. Recent large-scale prospective studies suggest that mediastinal enlargement in boys, and the presence of T-cell markers, indicate a poor prognosis, but the presence of a mediastinal mass without T-cell markers is not an indicator of poor prognosis.

5 *Total white cell count* Despite the use of intensive combination chemotherapy, the level of the white cell counts correlates most closely with prognosis. Patients with white cell counts less than 10×10^9/l have a significantly better prognosis than those with white cell counts between 10–100 $\times 10^9$/l. Patients with counts above 100×10^9/l have the worst prognosis. Even when patients with T-cell leukaemia are excluded from remission analysis, there is a significantly higher early relapse rate in patients with white cell counts over 100×10^9/l.

6 *Platelet counts* greater than 100×10^9/l at diagnosis appear to have a significantly higher total remission rate.

7 *Leukaemic CNS infiltration* at presentation is always a poor prognostic sign.

8 *Leukaemia cells surface markers* By the currently available techniques, it is possible to distinguish certain surface markers which relate the leukaemic cells to two subgroups of normal lymphocytes:

(a) 'T' (thymus) cell markers can be detected by rosetting with sheep red cells or by specific anti-T sera. The presence of T-cell markers occurs in approximately 10–20% of patients with leukaemia and indicate a poor prognosis.

(b) 'B' (bursa) cell markers may be detected by indirect immunofluorescence or immunoenzyme techniques for IgG on the surface of the cells or in the cytoplasm. They occur in less than 1% of patients with ALL and indicate the worst prognosis.

In the majority, there are no markers on the cell surface which relate the leukaemia cells to a normal lymphocyte cell population. These patients have the best prognosis. Recently, some workers have presented evidence that these cells have differentiation antigens which distinguish them from normal mature lymphocytes. Approximately 80% of patients with ALL react with sera raised to these differentiation antigens and have been called 'common ALL'. They respond best to treatment. The remainder of the patients who are T- and B-cell negative and have no differentiation antigens detectable with currently available antibodies, have been termed 'null cell' ALL and do not respond as well to treatment as do the 'common' type.

9 *Enzyme markers* It has been shown that acid phosphatase levels are specifically elevated in T-cell leukaemia and that high acid phosphatase levels correlate with poor prognosis. This has not been confirmed in recent studies. Terminal deoxynucleotidyl transferase (TdT) activity is significantly raised in ALL as compared to other leukaemias. No significant differences in TdT have been found in patients with T-cell leukaemia and the level of TdT does not correlate with prognosis. Similarly, there is no association between prognosis and the labelling or mitotic index or bone marrow culture characteristics.

Management

This can be considered under the following headings: (1) remission induction, (2) intensification, (3) CNS prophylaxis, (4) continuation chemotherapy and (5) discontinuation of treatment.

REMISSION INDUCTION

Before commencing chemotherapy, an adequate urine output should be induced with intravenous fluids. Uric acid nephropathy may be prevented by ensuring a high urinary flow, alkalinization of the urine and administration of allopurinol 10 mg/kg for 24 hours prior to commencing chemotherapy. In some patients with massive organomegaly and very high white cell counts, it may be useful to lower the tumour cell mass by leukophoresis on a cell separator prior to chemotherapy.

The most commonly used induction programmes use vincristine, prednisolone and asparaginase. An alternative consists of vincristine and prednisolone only or the addition of an anthracycline such as daunorubicin or adriamycin. Controlled studies have shown that in the usual patient with

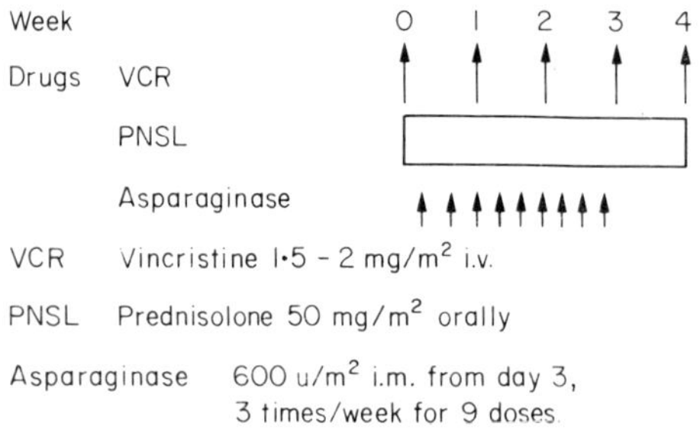

Fig. 7.4 The asparaginase induction schedule tested by the Children's Cancer Study Group.

ALL, there is no increased incidence of remission induction when anthracyclines are combined with vincristine and prednisolone, but the effect of anthracyclines during induction on the length of complete remission has not been defined. The addition of asparaginase to the induction programme increases the length of complete remission, particularly when asparaginase is administered after commencing vincristine and prednisolone. Remission induction rates with multiple drugs in ALL range from 85 to 97%. A representative induction schedule using asparaginase and tested in large numbers of patients by Children's Cancer Study Group, is shown in Fig. 7.4.

INTENSIFICATION

There has been much argument about the value of intensification phases of treatment following remission induction. There is no conclusive evidence that intensification therapy is of value. In studies performed at St Jude Children's Research Hospital, intensification, using intravenous 6-mercaptopurine, methotrexate and cyclophosphaemide, did not prolong the duration of remission and, to date, there are no controlled studies from other centres that show it to be of value. Another approach used by the Sidney Farber Cancer Institute has been to assess the response to remission induction therapy by the use of bone marrow aspiration after 3 weeks of treatment and to administer intensification therapy such as vincristine 2 mg/m^2 i.v. on day 1, adriamycin 35 mg/m^2 i.v. on day 1, 6-mercaptopurine 225 mg/m^2 orally daily for 5 days, followed by L-asparaginase 30 000–60 000 u/m^2 i.m. or i.v. for 2–4 doses. Other schemes, such as the one under investigation at the Sloan Kettering Memorial Hospital, use three alternating course of intravenous methotrexate followed by cytosine arabinoside and 6-thioguanine, followed by asparaginase and high dose cyclophosphamide.

PRESYMPTOMATIC CNS THERAPY

Primary CNS relapse terminated remission in more than 60% of children when no specific treatment was directed for the prevention of symptomatic CNS infiltration. Pioneering studies at St Jude Children's Research Hospital have unequivocally demonstrated that CNS therapy with 2400 rad cranial irradiation and five injections of intrathecal methotrexate at intervals of 1 week, soon after induction of remission and before there is clinical and laboratory evidence of CNS infiltration, can reduce the incidence of CNS leukaemia to about 5–10%. The role of presymptomatic CNS therapy is now established beyond doubt, but it is uncertain what mode of therapy is most effective. Intrathecal chemotherapy given as a single course has clearly been shown to be ineffective. Some centres claim that presymptomatic CNS therapy with regular injections of intrathecal chemotherapy, together with the use of the nitrosoureas during maintenance, produce results which are as good as those with cranial irradiation and five intrathecal injections of methotrexate.

In one controlled study, it has been demonstrated that cranial irradiation to 1800 rad is as effective as 2400 rad with adequate long-term follow-up. These questions remain unresolved, as no randomized controlled studies with an adequate duration of follow-up comparing these regimens have yet been published. As a reasonable compromise, many centres are administering initial cranial irradiation of 1800 rad and intrathecal methotrexate as well as maintenance intrathecal methotrexate every 8–18 weeks.

CONTINUATION THERAPY

It is clearly established that continuation therapy is necessary in ALL and that multiple drug continuation is superior to single drug therapy. Although many centres incorporate short periods of reinduction in the programme of continuation therapy, there is no evidence that this significantly prolongs the duration of remission or survival. There is a general tendency to use intermittent rather than continuous chemotherapy, as this reduces the degree of immunosuppression and opportunistic infections. Centres using intermittent continuation chemotherapy report results which are at least as good as those with continuous chemotherapy but, as yet, no randomized study comparing these two methods of continuation chemotherapy has been published. There is also no evidence that continuation therapy utilizing multiple drugs in a cyclic manner is superior to regimens which use the same drugs continuously or in repeated cycles.

The following are some of the simpler schedules of continuation therapy which are well established:

Continuous treatment

6-Mercaptopurine 50–75 mg/m^2 orally daily
methotrexate 20–30 mg/m^2 i.v., i.m. or orally weekly.

Continuous treatment plus reinduction

6-Mercaptopurine and methotrexate as above with reinduction using vincristine i.v., prednisolone orally and asparaginase i.m. every 3–6 months.

Repeated use of the same drugs in cycles (As an example, the Sidney Farber Cancer Institute protocol for ALL is shown)

Vincristine 2 mg/m^2 day 1 i.v.
adriamycin 30 mg/m^2 day 1 i.v.
6-mercaptopurine 225 mg/m^2 day 1–5 orally
prednisolone 120 mg/m^2 day 1–5 orally
Cycle repeated every 14–21 days.

DISCONTINUATION OF TREATMENT

There is no evidence that continuing anti-leukaemic treatment indefinitely can prevent late relapses and deaths from leukaemia. Randomized studies in which treatment is continued for 24 months beyond 3 years or discontinued at 3 years show no statistically significant difference in relapse rates, except for testicular relapses which occur more commonly in those boys who discontinue treatment at 3 years. These studies are not entirely randomized, as families of the children with ALL may elect to continue or discontinue treatment.

When therapy is discontinued after 19 months of complete remission, there is a significantly higher incidence of bone marrow relapse than in patients who continue treatment for a further 18 months.

Various studies of large numbers of patients (St Jude Hospital Children's Cancer Study Group) have shown that the continuous remission rate after stopping treatment is approximately 80%. At the present time in the majority of centres, treatment ceases after 2.5–3 years of total remission. Many, but not all, centres are reporting a disturbingly high incidence of testicular relapse in boys discontinuing treatment. At the time of discontinuation of treatment, bone marrow aspiration, lumbar puncture and bilateral testicular biopsies should be performed to ensure that the patient is truly in remission.

Remission rates according to prognostic criteria

It is generally agreed that the overall expectation of leukaemia-free survival after 3 years of therapy is about 50%.

In patients with neither T- nor B-cell leukaemia treated by the methods previously outlined, 60–70% of children with white cell counts below $20–50 \times 10^9/l$ may be expected to be in remission after 3 years of continuation chemotherapy. In patients with high white cell counts, the proportion in remission is reduced to 40–50%.

In patients with T-cell leukaemia, the total remission rate after 2 years is usually reported to be between 10–30%. Children with B-cell leukaemia, or those under the age of 1 year, have an even worse prognosis than those with T-cell leukaemia.

Immunotherapy

Various forms of immunotherapy have been attempted. These include BCG alone, BCG and allogeneic cells, or mixtures of allogeneic cells, BCG and C. parvum or C. granulosum.

Only the group of workers from *Institut de Cancerologie et d'Immunogenetique* at Villejuif, France, has reported a beneficial effect from immunotherapy after 3–24 months of intensive chemotherapy and CNS prophylaxis. These results have not been confirmed by other studies where patients have been randomized to receive chemotherapy or immunotherapy after standard induction and optional CNS prophylaxis. A randomized study of intermittent chemotherapy ± BCG following induction and CNS prophylaxis, is currently in progress and shows no advantage for the BCG treated group. It is generally agreed that if immunotherapy has any role in the treatment of ALL, it will be as a relatively minor adjuvant to chemotherapy. This situation may alter when, or if, specific leukaemia antigens that can elicit an immune response can be isolated for therapeutic purposes.

Complications of treatment

A full description of these is not possible, but Table 7.2 summarizes those which are most common and require alertness to their possible occurrence so that they may be diagnosed rapidly and effectively treated.

Family and patient responses to the diagnosis and treatment of leukaemia and other malignancies

A diagnosis of leukaemia in a child is invariably a profound shock to the parents and other family members. In general, the response of the parent may be summarized as a sequence of several phases: anticipatory phase in which the worst is feared; a numbing impact phase when informed of the diagnosis; a recoil phase with depression, anxiety and uncertainty; a phase of mobilizing additional internal and external resources followed by a gradual readjustment

Table 7.2 Phases of leukaemic treatment and their complications.

Phase of leukaemic treatment	Complications
Induction	Uric acid nephropathy Septicaemia with Gram negative shock and DIC Hypocalcaemia or hypercalcaemia Transient diabetes mellitus Pancreatitis Idiosyncratic reaction to vincristine with inappropriate secretion of ADH and convulsions Acute haemorrhage due to thrombocytopenia ± hypo-prothrombinaemia
CNS prophylaxis	Postirradiation drowsiness Leucoencephalopathy (associated with moderate high-dose systemic methotrexate)
Continuation therapy	Overwhelming viral infections, e.g. measles, chickenpox or CMV Opportunistic infection, e.g. *Pneumocystis carinii*, methotrexate induced hepatic or pulmonary toxicity Cyclophosphamide induced haemorrhagic cystitis Pancytopenia and bacterial infections

to the new situation of requiring prolonged medical treatment and observation. Naturally, the response of individuals shows great variability. At all phases of treatment, it is best to be honest with parents, and it is essential to be prepared to repeat information. In general, children should be informed of their diagnosis and given an outline of treatment. In general, information is best conveyed by parents rather than medical or paramedical staff. When the child has come to know his or her doctor, then that person may be the best source of information.

The possibility of dying as the result of leukaemia should not be broached with the child during the early phases of therapy. In an occasional child, it may be necessary to discuss the possibility of dying if requested to do so by the child or parents. Children develop effective mechanisms of denial of imminent death and no purpose is served by breaking down these denials for the sake of being strictly honest with the child.

In the management of a family with leukaemia, it is wise to enlist the help of interested and experienced nursing staff, medical social workers and self-help groups. It is important that the staff looking after a child with leukaemia should maintain an air of optimism and confidence, even when staff members know the situation is hopeless. Despondency or depression among staff members saps the confidence and strength of the patients and their families.

Management of the dying child

Despite the great improvement in prognosis, 50% of patients still die from leukaemia. It is the role of the medical team to make death as painless and non-frightening as possible, and to allow it to take place within the family circle.

To achieve this, the following procedures are vital:

1 Alleviate pain with adequate analgesia.

Brompton cocktail, proladone suppositories (oxycodone pectinate) and intravenous morphine with chlorpromazine are usually effective in controlling pain.

Formula for Brompton cocktail

Morphine hydrochloride (or heroin) 15 mg
cocaine hydrochloride 10 mg
alcohol (90%) 2 ml
syrup 4 ml
chloroform water to 15 ml

In many children, cocaine may cause irritability and unpleasant hallucinations. In general, it should be omitted from the mixture.

Bone pain often responds poorly to analgesics and is best treated with intensive chemotherapy which may have to be administered in doses or timing which make it profoundly marrow toxic. Death from anaemia or occult haemorrhage is far preferable to persistent bone pain. Analgesia is often more effective in anaemic patients.

2 Prevent disabling infections with adequate antibiotic and other supportive therapy, which may include granulocyte transfusion. In particular, perineal lesions may cause the patients great discomfort and embarrassment.
3 Ensure that the child is not lonely by allowing them to be at home or, if this is impossible, by making adequate provisions for the child's parents to be with the child day and night. Siblings should be encouraged to visit frequently and to be involved in the anticipatory mourning process.
4 Avoid unnecessary investigations and painful procedures.
5 The child should receive optimal nursing and medical care, with regular visits from house and consultant staff.

ACUTE MYELOBLASTIC LEUKAEMIA (AML)

Under this term can be included other myeloblastic leukaemias with morphological features suggestive of greater differentiation (Table 7.1). The most important of these subgroups is acute promyelocytic leukaemia because it is often associated with disseminated intravascular coagulation.

Clinical presentation

Haemorrhagic symptoms are the most frequent mode of presentation. Less frequently, patients present with infections or bone pain. A peculiar, but rare, mode of presentation is periorbital infiltration giving rise to proptosis which may be associated with cranial nerve palsies. All ages may be involved, but, in childhood, the disease occurs more commonly in teenage or children under the age of 2 years. Sex distribution is even.

Clinical examination may lead to the suspicion of AML rather than ALL if there are signs of disseminated intravascular coagulation such as substantial echymoses, bleeding from gums and nose and bleeding from skin puncture sites. Occasionally, skin or palate infiltrates which have a purple colour may be seen and these represent local leukaemic infiltration (chloromas). The degree of hepatosplenomegaly and lymphadenopathy are variable. The presence of massive splenomegaly should cause one to suspect that there may have been transformation from chronic myeloid leukaemia to its terminal acute leukaemic phase, but this can only be confirmed by laboratory investigations.

Diagnosis

This is established by bone marrow aspiration. The morphological feature of AML may need to be confirmed by histochemical and enzyme investigations. Myeloblasts are usually Sudan black B and peroxidase positive and PAS negative. The terminal deoxynucleotidyl transferase level is low. Chromosome analysis frequently shows associated abnormalities, e.g. *t*(8:21);

addition of a number 8; loss of number 7. The occurrence of transformation from chronic myeloid leukaemia is confirmed by demonstration of the Philadelphia chromosome.

Prognostic features

Unlike ALL the likely prognosis cannot be assessed at the time of presentation. There is no close relationship between hepatosplenomegaly and total white cell count and the duration of remission or survival. Children with acute promyelocytic leukaemia are difficult to treat because of the associated DIC, but if they can be brought into remission, they may have prolonged survival. Children who have transformed from chronic myeloid leukaemia often fail to come into remission.

Prognosis

Complete remission can be induced in only 60–70% of children, irrespective of age. Patients who fail to come into remission usually die from toxicity of the induction treatment. The median duration of remission has been improved by vigorous induction chemotherapy with 70% of children still in remission at 12 months, but the median survival of all patients is still only approximately 12 months. It is uncertain whether patients with this disease can be cured, but plateaux of the remission and survival curves of approximately 20% at 30–36 months are now being reported.

Treatment

Vigorous chemotherapy to produce bone marrow aplasia is required to induce remission in a substantial proportion of patients. To achieve this aim, comprehensive supportive facilities are needed, including the availability of platelet and white cell transfusions. The mainstays of chemotherapy are cytosine arabinoside (Ara-C) and the anthracyclines. In general, Ara-C is given as a continuous infusion for 4–7 days (100–150 mg/m^2), and this is followed by daunomycin 30–50 mg/m^2 given daily for 2–3 days. A second course of chemotherapy should be administered as soon as practicable, usually 8–14 days after completion of the first. The presence of remission should be ascertained by marrow aspiration after 1–3 courses of chemotherapy. If partial remission is present, further chemotherapy, introducing other drugs such as intermittent courses of Ara-C with 6-thioguanine and cyclophosphamide and adriamycin may be of value.

The roles of maintenance chemotherapy and CNS prophylaxis remain debatable. There is no doubt that CNS infiltration occurs in AML in 10–15% of patients who survive for more than 6 months. In the author's unit, and increasingly more commonly in other units, CNS prophylaxis with intermittent intrathecal Ara-C (30 mg/m^2) is given after a fully documented remission has been attained.

There are no adequate studies which prove that remission maintenance prolongs the duration of survival or remission. Nevertheless, in the majority of centres, patients are given remission maintenance in the form of intermittent chemotherapy using Ara-C and 6-thioguanine. There is some evidence that immunotherapy with adjuvants such as BCG or MRE, together with allogeneic cells, may prolong the duration of survival but adequately randomized studies on large numbers of patients are lacking.

DIC

DIC occurs most often in promyelocytic leukaemia and may be present before treatment has commenced or after chemotherapy. Its management requires the use of heparin and infusions of coagulation factor concentrates, platelets and fresh frozen plasma as a source of antithrombin III. It is the author's practice to administer low dose heparin (100 u/kg/24 h) and fresh frozen plasma before commencing chemotherapy, in an attempt to augment functional antithrombin III activity. If DIC develops during treatment, the dose of heparin is increased to 400–600 u/kg/24 h, and platelet and co-agulation factor concentrates are infused.

CHRONIC MYELOID LEUKAEMIA

The adult type of CML, with Philadelphia chromosome (*t* (9:22) translocation of part of the distal long arms of chromosome 22 to chromosome 9), presents with marked hepatosplenomegaly and a leucocytosis usually without anaemia or thrombocytopenia. Marrow aspiration shows gross myeloid hyperplasia and plentiful megakaryocytes. The condition may respond to treatment with a standard (0.06 mg/kg daily orally) or high dose (75 mg/m^2 single oral dose) of myleran, but is usually more difficult to treat than its adult counterpart. If daily myleran is used, the dose must be lowered when a fall of the total white cell count has occurred after 2–4 weeks of treatment and myleran should be discontinued when the white cell count reaches levels of 20 000. Conversion to acute myeloid leukaemia or, more rarely, acute lymphocytic leukaemia occurs regularly within 1–3 years from presentation. This constitutes one of the strongest lines of evidence that haemopoietic precursors and lymphoid cells may share a common pluripotential stem cell. Patients who transform to acute lymphocytic leukaemia usually respond well to chemotherapy, but have only short remissions. Transformation to acute myeloid leukaemia is very difficult to treat, as it responds poorly to the usual chemotherapy used for the treatment of acute myeloblastic leukaemia.

JUVENILE CHRONIC MYELOID LEUKAEMIA

This appears to be a myeloproliferative disorder. Patients present with hepatosplenomegaly, with predominant enlargement of the spleen and often a facial rash described as eczematous or pustular. There is a variable increase in white cell count, marked anaemia and thrombocytopenia. The bone marrow shows myeloid proliferation with decrease in erythroid precursors and megakaryocytes. The fetal Hb level is often markedly increased, and there may be other fetal characteristics such as low Hb/A_2 and unusual surface *i* antigen. Chromosome analysis does not show a Philadelphia chromosome, though other abnormalities, particularly in Groups 21 and 22, have been described. Patients do not respond well to treatment with myleran or 6-mercaptopurine or the type of therapy used for acute myeloblastic leukaemia. A splenectomy may be required to alleviate discomfort and pain from a grossly enlarged spleen.

VERY RARE CHILDHOOD LEUKAEMIAS

Monocytic leukaemia

A true monocytic leukaemia is differentiated from the more common myelomonocytic variety by the presence of predominantly monocytes and monoblasts on the peripheral blood film and bone marrow aspiration, and by raised urine muramidase levels and strong staining for alpha naphthyl acetate esterase. Clinically, patients with monocytic leukaemia may show marked gum hypertrophy, lymphadenopathy and features of DIC. The treatment is as for acute myeloblastic leukaemia. The new epipodophylotoxin VP16 appears to be a promising drug for monocytic leukaemia. Patients usually respond well to treatment and prolonged survivals are well documented. CNS infiltration is common in patients with prolonged survival and CNS prophylaxis may be of value.

Histiocytic leukaemia

Occasionally, patients with histiocytic lymphoma may have circulating histiocytic cells and marrow infiltration with cells whose morphological features resemble those of histiocytic lymphoma cells. Sometimes, there is no primary focus of lymphoma, but the patients present with pancytopenia and bone marrow infiltration. These patients usually respond well to treatment with chemotherapy programmes which include anthracyclines. In the author's experience, CNS infiltration in histiocytic lymphoma is rare and it is doubtful whether these children require irradiation as a form of CNS prophylaxis.

Erythroleukaemia (Di-Guglielmo's syndrome)

A true erythroleukaemia is exceedingly rare in childhood. More commonly in acute myeloblastic leukaemia, there may also be erythroblastic proliferation.

Patients present with severe anaemia, thrombocytopenia and neutropenia. Bone marrow aspirate shows replacement by immature and morphologically abnormal erythroblasts. The condition may respond temporarily to treatment programmes which include as a main therapeutic agent, cytosine arabinoside.

BONE MARROW TRANSPLANTATION

In children with ALL who have relapsed and à second remission has been induced transplantation results in 30% long term disease free survival rates. At the present time, transplantation can only be undertaken if there are HLA and mixed lymphocyte culture compatible sibling donors. Recurrence of leukaemia, despite whole body irradiation and high dose cyclophaphamide, and graft versus host disease are the main complications. In AML transplantation during first remission results in 50–70% long term disease-free survival rates. Graft versus host disease but not recurrence of leukaemia is the major complication.

RECOMMENDED READING

Cell kinetics and theoretical models of treatment

Mauer A.M., Evert C.F.J., Lampkin B.C. et al. (1973) Cell kinetics in human acute lymphoblastic leukaemia: computer simulation with descrete modelling techniques. *Blood* **41**, 141.

Mauer A.M. (1975) Cell kinetics and practical consequences for therapy of acute leukemia. *New England Journal of Medicine* **293**, 389.

Murphy S.B., Aur R.J.A., Simone J.V., George S. & Mauer A.M. (1977) Pretreatment cytokinetic studies in 94 children with acute leukemia. Relationship to other variables at diagnosis and to outcome of standard treatment. *Blood* **49**, 683.

General aspects and clinical features of infections

Bodey G.P., Rodriguez V., Chang H.-Y. & Narboni G. (1978) Fever and infection in leukemic patients. A study of 494 consecutive patients. *Cancer* **41**, 1610.

Gurwith M.J., Brunton J.L., Lank B.A., Harding G.K.M. & Ronald A.R. (1979) A prospective controlled investigation of prophylactic trimethoprim/sulfamethoxazole in hospitalized granulocytogenic patients. *American Journal of Medicine* **66**, 284.

Lascari A.D. (1973) *Leukemia in Childhood,* Chapters 1, 2 & 7. Charles C. Thomas, Springfield, Illinois.

O'Regan S., Carson S., Chesney R.W. & Drummond K.N. (1977) Electrolyte and acid-base disturbances in the management of leukemia. *Blood* **49**, 345.

Psychosocial aspects

Baker L.S. (1978) *You and Leukemia: a day at a time*. W.B. Saunders Company, Philadelphia.

Prognostic factors

Chessells J.M. (1979) Presentation and prognosis in childhood leukemia. In *Topics in Paediatrics; Haematology and Oncology*, p. 27. Pitman Medical, London.

Dow L.W., Borella L., Sen L., Aur R.J.A., George S.L., Mauer A.M. & Simone J.V. (1977) Initial prognostic factors and lymphoblasts erythrocyte rosette formation in 109 children with acute lymphoblastic leukemia. *Blood* **50**, 671.

Zippin C., Cutler S.J., Reeves W.J., Jr. & Lum D. (1971) Variation in survival among patients with acute lymphocytic leukemia. *Blood* **37**, 59.

Cell markers

Greaves M.F. (1979) Molecular phenotypes: A new perspective on diagnosis and classification of leukaemias. In *Topics in Paediatrics; Haematology and Oncology*, p. 36. Pitman Medical, London.

Treatment

Haghbin M., Tan C.T.C., Clarkson B.D., Mike V., Burchenal J.H. & Murphy L.M. (1975) Treatment of acute lymphoblastic leukemia in children with 'prophylactic' intrathecal methotrexate and intensive systemic chemotherapy. *Cancer Research* **35**, 807.

Haghbin M., Tan C.C., Clarkson B.D., Mike V., Burchenal J.H. & Murphy M.L. (1974) Intensive chemotherapy in children with acute lymphoblastic leukemia. *Cancer* **33**, 1491.

Hustu H.O., Aur R.J.A., Verzosa M.S., Simone J.V. & Pinkel D. (1973) Prevention of central nervous system leukemia by irradiation. *Cancer* **32**, 585.

Lascari A.D. (1973) *Leukemia in Childhood*, Chapter 12. Charles C. Thomas, Springfield, Illinois.

Ortega J.A., Nesbit M.E., Jr., Donaldson M.H., Hittle R.E., Weiner J., Karon M. & Hammond D. (1977) L-asparaginase, vincristine and prednisone for induction of first remission in acute lymphocytic leukemia. *Cancer Research* **37**, 535.

Sallan S.E., Camitta B.M., Cassady R., Nathan D.G. & Frei E. III (1978) Intermittent combination chemotherapy with adriamycin for childhood acute lymphoblastic leukemia: Clinical results. *Blood* **51**, 425.

Simone J.V., Aur R.J.A., Hustu O.H., Verzosa M. & Pinkel D. (1975) Combined modality therapy of acute lymphocytic leukemia. *Cancer* **35**, 25.

Thomas D.E., Sanders J.E., Flairnoy N., Johnson F.L., Buckner C.D., Clift R.A., Fefer A., Goodell B.W., Storb R. & Weiden P.L. (1979) Marrow transplantation for patients with acute lymphoblastic leukemia in remission. *Blood* **54**, 468.

Duration of treatment and results of cessation of treatment

BAUM E., SATHER H., NACHMAN J., SEINFELD J., KRIVIT W., LEIKIN S., MILLER D., JOO P. & HAMMOND D. (1979) Relapse rates following cessation of chemotherapy during complete remission of acute lymphocytic leukemia. *Medical and Pediatric Oncology* **7**, 25.

GEORGE S.J., AUR R.J.A., MAUER A.M. & SIMONE J.V. (1979) A reappraisal of the results of stopping therapy in childhood leukemia. *New England Journal of Medicine* **300**, 269.

REPORT TO THE MEDICAL RESEARCH COUNCIL BY THE WORKING PARTY ON LEUKEMIA IN CHILDHOOD (1977) Treatment of acute lymphoblastic leukemia: effect of variation in length of treatment on duration of remission. *British Medical Journal* **2**, 495.

Granulocytic leukaemias

ALTMAN A.J., PALMER C.G. & BAEHNER R.L. (1974) Juvenile 'chronic granulocytic' leukemia: A pamyelopathy with prominent monocytic involvement and circulating monocyte colony forming cells. *Blood* **43**, 341.

CHOI SUN-I. & SIMONE J.V. (1976) Acute nonlymphocytic leukemia in 171 children. *Medical and Pediatric Oncology* **2**, 119.

HAGHBIN M., MURPHY M.L. & TAN C.T.C. (1977) Treatment of acute nonlymphoblastic leukemia in children with a multiple-drug protocol. *Cancer* **40**, 1417.

HARDISTY R.M., SPEED D.E. & TILL M. (1964) Granulocytic leukemia in childhood. *British Journal of Haematology* **10**, 551.

PREISLER H.D., RUSTUM Y., HENDERSON E.S., BJORNSSON S., CREAVEN P.J., HIGBY D.J., FREEMAN A., GIOLINI S. & NAEHER C. (1979) Treatment of acute non-lymphocytic leukemia: Use of anthracycline-cytosine arabinoside induction therapy and comparison of two maintenance regimens. *Blood* **53**, 455.

THOMAS E.D., BUCKNER C.D., BANAJI M., CLIFT R.A., FEFER A., FLAIRNOY N., GOODELL B.W., HICKMAN R.O., LERNER K.G., NEIMAN P.E., SALE G.E., SANDERS J.E., SINGER J., STEVENS M., STORB R. & WEIDEN P.L. (1977) One hundred patients with acute leukemia treated by chemotherapy, total body irradiation, and allogeneic marrow transplantation. *Blood* **49**, 511.

Chapter 8
Deficiences of Immune and Neutrophil Function

The immune and related systems are highly integrated, interacting groups of cells and cell products. The underlying principle of the system is that an initial recognition event occurs which then triggers a number of amplification mechanisms. Amplification can happen at the level of the recognizing cell (antigen sensitive lymphocyte) so that that cell itself divides and matures to produce either soluble products from the B cell line (antibodies) or lymphokines from both B and T cells. Further amplification occurs following the effect of lymphokines on other lymphocytes and other cell types, particularly phagocytes. The action of antibody is amplified by its ability to activate complement, when fixed to the antigen which is to be recognized by cells of the lymphoid, neutrophil and macrophage/monocyte lines.

As shown in Fig. 8.1, the cells of the immune system are derived from lymphoid precursors which themselves are derived from bone marrow stem cells. The lymphoid precursors, in fetal life, go to either the thymus or bursa, where they are programmed to become T or B cells respectively. The T and B cells then leave the thymus and bursa and pass to the peripheral lymphoid tissue to await their contact with individual antigens. On contact with the

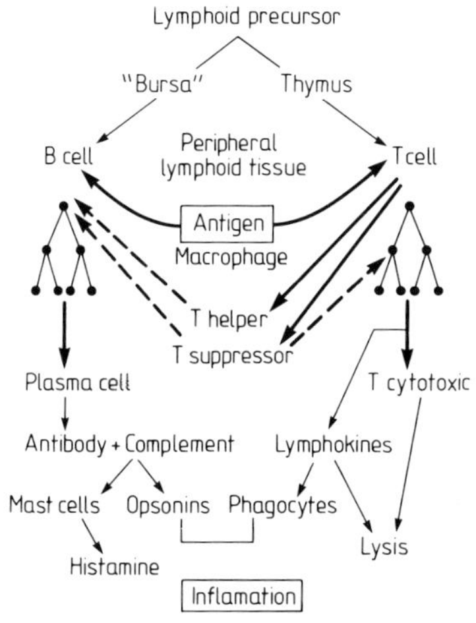

Fig. 8.1 Diagrammatic description of the derivation, functional development and amplification of the immune system.

antigen, there is initial triggering of cell division. This may result in the production of cytotoxic T cells and/or antibody secreting plasma cells.

The particular type of response elicited by an antigen is under the control of T cells which can help or suppress either wing of the immune system. While genetic influences are important, little is known of how the controls are set. After this recognition and initial specific amplification phase, the less specific amplification events of lymphokine action and complement activation occur.

The relative importance of many aspects of immune function have become apparent from the study of the rare, classical immune deficiency diseases. Much more common are secondary defects of immune function due either to other disease or their treatment with drugs that affect immune function. Because of the relatively non-specific action of drugs on the immune system, it is easier to gain knowledge of immune function by study of the immune deficiency diseases.

INFANTILE SEX-LINKED AGAMMAGLOBULINAEMIA

Clinical features

This was the first of the immune deficiency diseases described. Bruton, in 1953, reported on a boy of 7 years with a long history of life-threatening, bacterial infections. Investigation of his serum showed that he lacked gammaglobulin. Replacement of gammaglobulin by injection produced a marked improvement in his clinical state.

As implied in the name, this condition is found only in males, the female carriers are asymptomatic. Symptoms usually begin after 6 months of age as, until then, placentally transferred IgG prevents most infections. Until the diagnosis is made and replacement treatment instituted, these boys suffer from bacterial infections apparent in the respiratory tract and skin. It is important that the diagnosis be made early before permanent tissue damage, e.g. bronchiectasis, has occurred.

Diagnosis

The diagnosis should be suspected in any boy with the above symptoms. Serum electrophoresis confirms the lack of gammaglobulin, though further more detailed investigations are warranted to define the defect more accurately. Thus, quantitation of immunoglobulins of all major classes and examination of the surface membrane of lymphocytes for readily detectable immunoglobulin will help to categorize the patient more adequately and assist in genetic counselling.

Treatment

Treatment consists of intramuscular or intravenous gammaglobulin. The intramuscular preparation should not be given intravenously as it tends to fix complement and may cause severe reactions. The aim of treatment should be to maintain the level of IgG at greater than 28 i.u./ml (approximately 200 mg/100 ml) at all times.

Though there is individual variation in symptomatology unrelated to immunoglobulin levels at diagnosis, these boys can be kept reasonably free of infections on the above regimen. There is an increased incidence of auto-immune diseases and neoplasia in these patients.

THYMIC APLASIA

This abnormality was originally described by Di George, an endocrinologist who was investigating neonatal tetany. He found that, at post mortem, some of his patients had absent thymus glands, as well as parathyroids.

Clinical features

The disease is thought to be due to abnormalities of development of the third and fourth pharyngeal pouches, giving rise to the classical signs of:

1 Neonatal tetany.

2 Congenital heart disease, particularly affecting the great vessels at the base of the heart.

3 Recurrent infections in early infancy.

In the complete syndrome, there is a characteristic facies with hypertelorism, short upper lip philtrum and simple ear folds or deformed ears.

In the classical syndrome, these patients present initially with signs of congenital heart disease and neonatal tetany. Should the child survive these early problems, infections occur in the first few weeks or months of life. Often, these are fungal infections of the gastrointestinal tract and skin.

Diagnosis and treatment

The white cell count usually, but not invariably, reveals lymphopenia. More

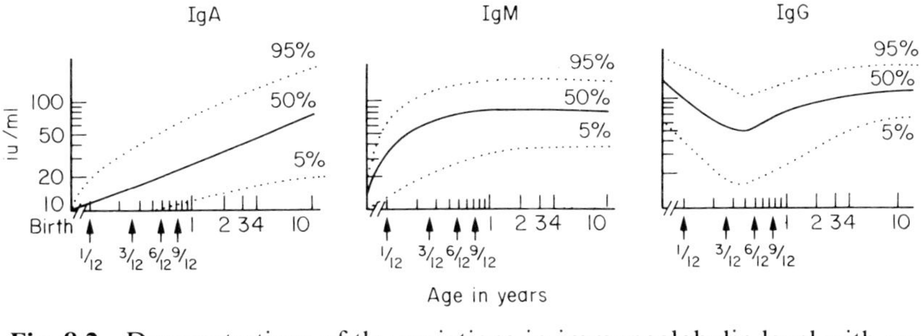

Fig. 8.2 Demonstrations of the variations in immunoglobulin level with age.

detailed immunological investigations show absence of lymphocytes able to form rosettes with sheep red cells (T cells) and an inability of lymphocytes to respond to T-cell mitogens. In some patients, fetal thymic transplant has been successful in restoring thymic function

Lesser degrees of the syndrome do occur and, at the present time, certainly some patients with apparent T-cell deficiency have been shown to have a deficiency of the enzyme, pyridine nucleotide phosphorylase. We shall have to wait to see the implications of these new findings.

SEVERE COMBINED IMMUNE DEFICIENCY

Originally called Swiss agammaglobulinaemia, after the nationality of the workers who described the syndrome, this disease is thought to be due to a lack of lymphoid precursor cells. These patients lack both T-cell and B-cell function. They have infections at an early age and, if the basic abnormality is uncorrected, usually die in the first year of life.

Diagnosis

Either sex can be affected and the disease is transmitted either in an autosomal recessive or sex-linked recessive mode. Approximately half of the children with the autosomal recessive form have a deficiency of the enzyme adenosine deaminase in their red cells and their parents have approximately half the normal levels of this enzyme. Diagnosis at an early age is important and should be considered in infants who develop watery diarrhoea, chest infections and fungal skin infections in the first few months of life. Investigation usually reveals lymphopenia and failure of lymphocytes to respond to mitogens. Serum immunoglobulins are usually, but not invariably, absent.

Treatment

In general, the only satisfactory long-term treatment for these infants is histocompatible bone marrow transplant. As a general rule, the donor should be an HLA matched, mixed lymphocyte reaction negative sibling. Care should be taken when transfusing these children. As these patients are unable to reject tissue grafts, the lymphocytes in normal blood recognize the patient as foreign and a graft versus host reaction may ensue. The blood should therefore be irradiated to prevent lymphocyte division.

To date, there are approximately 100 children around the world who have been treated with bone marrow transplantation, the majority of whom are doing well. The oldest child to have had such a transplant is now 13 years old.

If no histocompatible sibling is available, then the outlook is poor. Treatments that have been tried with variable degrees of success include fetal thymus transplant, cultured thymic epithelium transplant and fetal liver transplant.

ISOLATED IgA DEFICIENCY

Clinical significance

Isolated IgA deficiency is the commonest of the classical immune deficiency diseases. While the incidence of IgA deficiency in blood donor populations is approximately 1:700, it is much higher in populations of children with recurrent infections. We have estimated the incidence to be close to 5% in a population of children investigated for suspected immune deficiency. The implication from this is that while many otherwise healthy people are IgA deficient, IgA deficiency is significantly more common among children with recurrent infections. This may mean that on occasions IgA deficiency can be compensated for by other defence mechanisms or, alternatively, that in some people IgA deficiency is linked to another abnormality of immune function that predisposes to recurrent infections.

Treatment

Management of IgA deficiency depends entirely on the symptomatology. People with asymptomatic IgA deficiency do not require treatment. Patients with symptoms of recurrent infections and IgA deficiency may warrant a 3 month trial of intramuscular gammaglobulin. At the end of that time, a decision should be made, depending on the clinical response, as to whether or not to continue. While most gammaglobulin preparations contain only a trace of IgA, nevertheless it has been shown that there is often therapeutic benefit from such preparations.

IgA enriched gammaglobulin is also manufactured and, if the regular preparation fails to produce a positive response, then the IgA enriched gammaglobulin should be tried.

Miscellaneous

There are several other syndromes of immune deficiency in which the findings, clinically and immunologically, are not as clear cut as those above.

Ataxia telangiectasia a progressive cerebellar degenerative disease in which telangiectases are found on the bulbar conjunctiva, is accompanied by an immune deficiency which includes T-cell defects and, often, IgA deficiency. There is a high incidence of lymphoma.

The Wiskott-Aldrich syndrome is a sex-linked syndrome of eczema, thrombocytopenia, storage pool platelet function defect and susceptibility to infection. An inability to respond to polysaccharide antigens, including absent isohaemagglutinins, is another feature of the disease. There is a high incidence of lymphoma. Bone marrow transplantation from compatible siblings has been successful in the treatment of some children with this disorder.

Common variable immunodeficiency, largely unclassified

This constitutes the largest group of immune deficiencies, which were classified as such by the World Health Organisation. They form a heterogenous group, probably with a preponderance of patients with hypogammaglobulinaemia who do not fit any of the above classifications.

Neutrophil function defects

At the clinical level at the time of presentation, it may be quite difficult to distinguish a patient with a neutrophil defect from one with a classical immune deficiency.

CHRONIC GRANULOMATOUS DISEASE (CGD)

Pathogenesis and clinical features

CGD is the collective name for a number of defects of neutrophil oxidative metabolism that result in inability of neutrophils to be stimulated following ingestion of a micro-organism. The condition is usually inherited in a sex-linked recessive mode. The neutrophils have normal chemotaxis and phagocytocis, but, following ingestion of certain bacteria, there is failure of production of the products of oxidative metabolism (super-oxide and hydrogen peroxide) and resultant failure to kill the bacteria. To some extent, the defect is selective in that only bacteria that produce the enzyme, catalase, are able to survive within the neutrophil. This is because one of the major killing mechanisms within the phagocytic vacuole of the neutrophil is the combined action of myeloperoxidase, hydrogen peroxide and a halide — the iodination reaction. In CGD neutrophils, there is failure of hydrogen peroxide production. However, most bacteria produce some hydrogen peroxide. If the bacteria are catalase positive, then the bacterially produced hydrogen peroxide is broken down, and as the iodination reaction cannot take place in the absence of peroxide, the bacteria survive. Thus, most of the serious infections in children with chronic granulomatous disease are with catalase positive organisms. The clinical features are those of frequent infections, enlarged, occasionally suppurative, lymph nodes and leucocytocis. Non-resolving skin or pulmonary infections may be prominent features.

Treatment

There is some laboratory and considerable clinical evidence to suggest that patients with defects of neutrophil function are helped by treatment with sulpha drugs. The usual one used is either sulphafurazole or trimethoprim/ sulphamethoxazole.

INVESTIGATIONS OF CHILDREN WITH RECURRENT INFECTIONS

In general, there is a high incidence of infections in patients with diseases of both the lymphoid and granulocyte systems. The types of infecting micro-organisms that are associated with defects of antibody production and granulocyte function are the higher grade encapsulated organisms such as the *Streptococcus*, *Haemophilus influenzae*, *Pseudomonas aeruginosa* and *Pneumocystis carinii*. Cellular immune responses are important in limiting infections due to intracellular organisms such as viruses, mycobacteria and fungi.

Clinical approach

A clinician faced with a child with apparent recurrent infections needs to make two decisions. Firstly, is the child having infections and, if answered in the affirmative, are there host factors involved in the increased incidence of infections? In attempting to answer the first question, one should be aware of the possibility of allergic disease masquerading as infection. This is particularly so with 'upper respiratory infection' and 'bronchitis'. History, including family history and examination, may lead one to suspect this aetiology and simple tests, like a nasal smear for eosinophils and positive skin prick tests to common environmental allergens, may aid in making a decision. A therapeutic trial of antihistamines for 'URTI' or bronchodilators for 'bronchitis' may also help. If a decision cannot be made at that level, then investigations of immune and neutrophil function may be warranted.

The diagnosis of *fibrocystic disease* should always be thought of in a child presenting with recurrent chest infections. The possibility of milk inhalation, either because of *pharyngeal incoordination* or an *H-shaped tracheo-oesophageal fistula* should also be entertained in the younger child with infections.

If lung infection is localized to a distinct anatomical area, then the presence of a foreign body or anatomical defect should be excluded before proceeding with immune function tests.

Table 8.1 Suggested list of basic immunologic investigations.

Investigation	Normal range
Humoral immunity — serum immunoglobulins	
IgG	See Fig. 16.1
IgA	See Fig. 16.1
IgM	See Fig. 16.1
Cell mediated immunity	
Response to mitogens: PHA	H3T incorporation 0.6 μg/ml purified PHA H3T incorporation 0μg/ml purified PHA Median = 50; range 20–100
Neutrophil function tests	
Phagocytosis	Opsonins to Baker's yeast: phagocytic index Median = 3.5; range 2.0–5.5
Glucose oxidation	cpm stimulated cpm unstimulated
$^{14}CO_2$ production	Median = 3.0; range 2.3–7.5
NBT — qualitative	
— quantitative	OD 515 stimulated OD 515 unstimulated Median = 3.3; range 2.0–5.3
Neutrophil iodination	65–135% of mean of controls

All of these normal ranges need to be established for individual laboratories.

Table 8.2 Immunological disorders and their diagnostic abnormalities.

Disease	Diagnostic laboratory abnormality
Infantile sex-linked agammaglobulinaemia	Absent IgA, IgM. Greatly reduced IgG
Thymic aplasia	Lymphopenia: absent response to mitogens.
Severe combined immunodeficiency	Lymphopenia: reduced immunoglobulins and mitogen response ± adenosine deaminase deficiency
Isolated IgA deficiency	Absent IgA
Common variable immune deficiency	Reduced immunoglobulins and ± deficient mitogen response
Chronic Granulomatous Disease	Deficient NBT response. Stimulated $^{14}CO_2$ production from 1-^{14}C-glucose reduced. Deficient neutrophil iodination

Investigations

Most of the above diseases can be diagnosed on clinical features and appropriate investigations. If the above diseases can be excluded, then a history of recurrent infections warrants detailed immunological investigations. It should be remembered that many of these deficiencies are treatable and delay in diagnosis may result in permanent tissue damage. The clinical history and examination, as outlined above, will suggest which investigations may be most usefully performed. In Table 8.1 are set out a list of comprehensive investigations which should be used to confirm the diagnosis of the suspected immunologic disorder. In Table 8.2 are listed the immunologic disorders and the associated diagnostic abnormality.

RECOMMENDED READING

HAYWARD A.R. (1977) *Immunodeficiency. Current Topics in Immunology.* Edward Arnold, London.

MIMS C.A. (1977) *The Pathogenesis of Infectious Diseases.* Academic Press, London.

ROITT I. (1980) *Essential Immunology*, 4th edn. Blackwell Scientific Publications, London.

Chapter 9
Iron Deficiency Anaemia

Normal values and definition of anaemia

Shortly after birth the haemoglobin levels range from 17 to 21 g/dl, the packed cell volume (PCV) from 54 to 68% and the red cells are macrocytic with a mean cell volume (MCV) of 119 μ^3. Subsequently there is a rapid drop in all values, so that by 2 months after birth the mean haemoglobin is 11 g/dl, the PCV 33% and the MCV 95 μ^3. Thereafter the haemoglobin and PCV values rise gradually to a level of 12–14 g/dl by 10 years of age. Adult haemoglobin levels are achieved at the time of puberty. In general after 8 weeks of life significant anaemia can be considered to be present if the haemoglobin level is below 10 g%.

IRON METABOLISM

The red cell is a non-nucleated cell with the sole function of carrying oxygen from the lungs to the body tissues and carbon dioxide from the tissues to the lungs. Approximately 3 000 000 red cells are produced in the bone marrow each second to replace those which die at the end of their 120 day life span. Production of the red cell is under the control of many factors. The DNA coding for the production of messenger RNA must be intact. Ribosomes, mitochondria, enzyme systems, an adequate supply of amino-acids, sugars, iron and other trace metals must all be available for adequate production. The rate of red cell production is influenced by a number of hormones, including erythropoietin and the hormones of the thyroid, pituitary and adrenal glands. Energy must be available to the red cell from the breakdown of glucose, provided by the enzymes of the Embden-Meyerhof pathway and the Pentose Phosphate pathway. Abnormalities in any one of the numerous factors involved in the production or maintenance of red cell function will result in decreased production or early destruction. Of all these factors iron deficiency, due to either poor diet, poor absorption or excessive bleeding, is the commonest cause of anaemia. Haemoglobin contains 65% of the body stores of iron. It is a complex molecule, composed of two pairs of dissimilar globin chains with one molecule of haem attached to each chain. Haemoglobin constitutes 99% of the red cell protein and its sole purpose is the transport of oxygen to tissues and carbon dioxide away from the tissues. Myoglobin is a similar compound to haemoglobin, but contains only one molecule of globin coupled to one haem molecule. It is the red pigment of muscle and stores the oxygen for use by the muscle during contraction. It contains less than 5% of the body iron stores.

At birth, the iron content of the body is related to weight. In the newborn, it is 75 mg of iron/kg body weight, and increases to 3–5 g in the adult. The iron is distributed into two compartments: (1) metabolic and enzyme iron and (2) storage and transport iron.

Metabolic iron and enzyme iron

Haemoglobin contains 65% of the body iron stores. Haemoglobin is a compound of four globin chain with one haem molecule attached. Myoglobin is the red pigment in muscle and is present in concentrations of 1–3 mg per gram of muscle tissue. Its function is to store the oxygen for muscle use.

The cytochromes contain around 1% of the body iron and are enzymes found in the mitochondria of cells and in cellular membranes. They are involved in electron transport and are necessary for the production of ATP.

Catalases and peroxidases contain small amounts of iron, are widely distributed in tissues and are involved in the reduction of endogenously produced H_2O_2.

Storage and transport

Iron is stored as a ferric-protein complex, equally divided between liver, bone marrow, spleen and reticuloendothelial tissue. The main storage proteins are ferritin and haemosiderin.

Ferritin is a compound of 24 identical units of protein with a central core of colloidal ferric phosphate. Iron makes up approximately 25% of the molecule. It does not stain with potassium ferrocyanide.

Haemosiderin has a less well defined molecular structure and is probably a heterogeneous group of compounds. It contains about 30% iron and stains for iron with potassium ferrocyanide.

Transferrin is the plasma iron transport protein; it is a globulin and is made in the liver. Each molecule of transferrin is capable of binding two molecules of ferric iron. It transports iron from the gut or the site of metabolism to the bone marrow, where the ferric ions are released for re-utilization to form haem, or for storage in the reticuloendothelial tissue.

Iron stores

At birth, 75% of the iron is present in the circulating haemoglobin, while the remainder is in the storage and enzyme pools. Total body iron stores at birth are affected by the blood volume, which may vary from 70 to 100 ml/kg body weight. Early clamping of the cord or milking blood from the placenta will profoundly affect the iron stores.

The presence of iron deficiency in the mother does not appear to result in iron deficiency anaemia in the newborn. Birth weight, rate of growth, iron supplementation or blood loss play a far more important role in the development of iron deficiency.

The stores present at birth in the mature infant are sufficient for about 4 months of normal requirements. From 4 months to 1 year, about 200 mg of iron are required for production of haem and for normal growth (0.8 mg/day). To supply these needs, a daily oral intake of at least 1 mg/kg/day of elemental iron must occur, assuming an absorption efficiency of around 10%.

Absorption

DIETARY FACTORS

Dietary iron is found mainly in meats, fish and in some green vegetables. Gut absorption occurs mainly in the duodenum, as the pH and redox potential are favourable in this site. Absorption occurs throughout the gut, but decreases progressively in the more distal parts.

Between 5 and 10% of the iron in the diet is usually absorbed. While the proportion absorbed decreases with increasing iron ingestion, the total amount absorbed is increased. Meat iron is absorbed better than vegetable iron, being as high as 20–30% for liver and red meat, and less than 5% for eggs, corn, spinach and wheat. Breast and cow's milk contain only small amounts of iron (0.5–1.5 mg/l) and contribute less than 5% of the recommended intake.

There are two forms of iron in food: haem iron and non-haem iron. The absorption of haem iron (haemoglobin, myoglobin) is different from non-haem iron. The haem is split from its apoprotein by gastric hydrochloric acid and proteases. On entering the mucosal cell, the iron is split from the porphyrin. The iron is then absorbed into the plasma in the same fashion as ionic iron. The absorption of haem iron is independent of the body iron balance.

Non-haem iron in food exists mainly in the form of ferric complexes. The iron is released from the ferric complexes by the action of gastric hydrochloric acid and organic acids. It is then reduced to the ferrous form by reducing substances such as ascorbic acid, fructose, lactate and sulphydryl groups in proteins. There are inhibitory effects exerted by phytates present in food because of the formation of insoluble salts with iron. Pancreatic juices also appear to inhibit absorption, possibly because of their alkaline pH.

MUCOSAL FACTORS

Iron is absorbed rapidly at the brush border of the mucosal cell in the crypts of Lieberkühn. At low levels of iron, the transfer is active and is dependent on the divalent state of iron and oxidative metabolism. At higher luminal concentrations of iron, there is also passive diffusion. A proportion of the iron passes into the plasma within a few hours. The remainder is incorporated into mucosal ferritin. This ferritin iron is lost when the cell is shed after 3–4 days.

By this mechanism, there is some regulation of iron absorption. In iron deficiency states, most of the absorbed iron is transferred to the plasma, while the mucosal cells retain little of the iron. During iron overload, a smaller proportion of the iron is taken up into the mucosal cell, that taken up being bound to ferritin which is subsequently lost when the mucosal cell is shed.

Control mechanisms governing the amount of iron absorbed are not clear. Increased absorption occurs during iron deficiency, dyserythropoietic states (thalassaemia, sideroblastic anaemia), anoxia, with increased erythropoiesis (following haemorrhage, haemolytic anaemia) and during pregnancy. It has been suggested that absorption may be regulated by the plasma iron level, by the percentage iron saturation of transferrin, or the rate of iron turnover. These cannot be the sole factors, as iron overload occurs with congenital absence of transferrin. It is thought that the haemoglobin level, hypoxia or erythropoietin do not have any direct effect on the mucosal cells.

IRON DEFICIENCY ANAEMIA

Iron deficiency anaemia is the commonest cause of anaemia, both in children and in adults. In children under the age of 5 years, a deficiency of iron in the diet is the most frequent cause of the anaemia, while blood loss is a less common cause. Rarely, malabsorption due to chronic diarrhoea or inflammatory bowel disease may be the cause of iron deficiency.

Aetiology

DIETARY

Symptoms of inadequate intake of iron due to faulty diet manifest themselves after the age of 4 months, a time when iron stores are depleted. In premature infants iron stores are depleted earlier and iron deficiency may manifest by the age of 1–2 months. Excessive intake of milk and carbohydrate is a common cause of dietary iron deficiency in affluent sections of the community. Dietary fads, including prolonged breast feeding without a complementary diet, are also becoming common causes of iron deficiency. In poor communities, inadequate caloric intake, high consumption of cereals and, frequently, parasitic infestation lead to iron deficiency.

GROWTH

Factors such as low birth weight (prematurity, twin pregnancy) and the growth spurt of puberty influence the need for iron and may result in iron deficiency.

Prematurity is almost invariably associated with iron deficiency, even when a normal diet is given to the child, and iron supplementation is required for all premature babies.

BLOOD LOSS

This can be considered in two categories: perinatal and postnatal.

Perinatal

1 Fetomaternal haemorrhage.
2 Retroplacental loss.
3 Placenta praevia.
4 Fetofetal haemorrhage.
5 Rupture of the cord.
6 Bleeding from the cord due to inadequate tying.
7 Inadequate replacement of blood following exchange transfusion.

Postnatal

1 Intestinal bleeding may occur at any site. This may be overt or occult and either acute or chronic. Causes vary and include:
(a) oesophageal varices.
(b) peptic and oesophageal ulceration.
(c) ingestion of aspirin or steroids.
(d) bleeding due to ectopic gastric mucosa in a Meckel's diverticulum.
(e) parasitic infestations, e.g. hookworm.
(f) ulcerative colitis.
(g) recurrent gastroenteritis.
(h) iron deficiency can of itself be accompanied by chronic blood loss associated with mucosal atrophy.
(i) milk allergy — this remains a controversial topic. There is little doubt that a well documented allergy to milk proteins can be associated with gastrointestinal blood loss leading to iron deficiency. Such patients are rare. Opinion remains sharply divided as to whether the child with unexplained iron deficiency and no firm evidence of milk allergy may have gastrointestinal blood loss due to exposure of gut mucosa to milk proteins. The condition appears to be more commonly described in the USA than in other parts of the world.
(j) congenital bleeding disorders, e.g. haemophilia, von Willebrand's disease, hereditary haemorrhagic telangiectasia.

2 Lung — Pulmonary haemosiderosis and Goodpastures syndrome may present as iron deficiency.
3 Malabsorption — Coeliac disease may present with iron deficiency after the age of one year.

Pathogenesis

When the body enters a negative iron balance, first call is made on tissue stores for the iron required for haemoglobin formation. When these stores are depleted, the synthesis of haemoglobin falls, resulting in the appearance of small red cells with low haemoglobin content (microcytic hypochromic anaemia).

Clinical features

There is usually a gradual onset of symptoms and signs. Pallor is often first noted by persons outside the family and is often accompanied by irritability in the child, anorexia and lethargy. Food fadism may occur, with the ingestion of dirt, stones and substances of no nutritional value (pica). An increased tendency to infections may be noted.

Physical examination

The child may appear undernourished. Pallor of the mucous membranes or the skin is noted. Occasionally there is slight enlargement of the spleen. If severe anaemia exists, there may be cardiomegaly and a soft apical systolic murmur may be present.

Laboratory investigations

There is a reduced haemoglobin level and the haematocrit is low, the MCHC is below 30%, MCV is less than 80 fl, and the MCH below 29 pg. The blood film shows microcytosis and hypochromia, with some anisocytosis and poikilocytes (pencil cells). Reticulocytes are reduced in number, unless iron has been recently administered or there has been recent haemorrhage.

Bone marrow examination shows erythroid hyperplasia with a predominance of the mature erythroblasts. The cytoplasm is reduced in amount and has a ragged outline, while the nucleus is small and deep staining (micronormoblastic erythropoiesis). Staining for iron with potassium ferrocyanide fails to show any iron stores. Bone marrow aspiration is seldom necessary to make the diagnosis, but may be necessary to exclude other causes of hypochromic anaemia.

Serum iron levels are reduced below the lower limit of normal (9 μm mol/1), serum iron binding capacity is raised and the percentage transferrin saturation is reduced. The serum ferritin level is reduced to below 12 ng/ml and the erythrocyte protoporphyrin is raised above the upper limit of normal (40 ng/dl erythrocytes).

Differential diagnosis

The diagnosis of iron deficiency anaemia is usually obvious and can be readily confirmed by noting correction of the anaemia in response to oral iron therapy. Occasionally, more sophisticated investigations may be required. A list of other conditions which may mimic iron deficiency anaemia and the critical investigations which confirm their existences, is shown in Table 9.1.

Table 9.1 Conditions which may mimic iron deficiency anaemia.

Condition	Critical diagnostic test
Thalassaemia and haemoglobinopathies	Hb electrophoresis*
Sideroblastic anaemia	Ringed sideroblasts on bone marrow aspiration seen after staining for iron Normal or high serum iron
Chemically induced anaemias, e.g. lead poisoning	Serum and tissue lead levels
Altransferrinaemia	Reduced or absent serum transferrin
Copper deficiency	Reduced copper levels
Chronic infections	Raised serum ferritin, reduced serum iron and total iron binding capacity

*Note that coexisting iron deficiency may cause the level of HbA_2 to be reduced to normal. The test should be repeated after correction of the iron deficiency.

Treatment

The presence of anaemia indicates that body stores of iron are depleted and treatment with iron should be continued for 3 months after the haemoglobin has been restored to normal values. The following principles should be followed.

1 Find and correct the causes of blood loss.

2 Correct dietary deficiencies. Introduce meat, eggs and vegetables to the diet. Limit milk to no more than one litre per day.

3 Administer oral iron. Oral iron is administered as the ferrous salt. Ferrous sulphate, ferrous gluconate and ferrous succinate are commonly used. Ferrous sulphate mixture is unstable, so that ferrous gluconate mixture is recommended. Tablets of all forms are available.

Prophylactic dose 2 mg elemental iron/kg/day in three divided doses between meals.

Therapeutic dose 6 mg elemental iron/kg/day in three divided doses between meals.

100 mg of ferrous sulphate is equivalent to 20 mg of elemental iron; 100 mg of ferrous gluconate is equivalent to 11 mg of elemental iron.

Oral iron may be administered with meals or before meals with orange juice. Milk and cereal products should be avoided if oral iron preparations are given. Occasionally, patients suffer side effects from oral iron, e.g. epigastric pain, nausea, diarrhoea and constipation. These patients may respond to a change of the iron preparation to a chelated iron preparation, e.g. Plesmet.

4 Parenteral iron. Occasionally parenteral iron is administered because of factors such as diarrhoea, refusal to take oral iron by the child, non-compliance by the parents, Malabsorption syndrome, severe anaemia (Hb < 5 g%) and intolerance to any form of oral iron therapy. Iron may be given by the intramuscular route or by infusion.

The total amount of elemental iron required in milligrams is calculated as follows:

$$\frac{\text{Normal Hb for age} - \text{patient's Hb}}{100} \times \text{blood volume (ml)} \times 3.4 \times 1.5.$$

The blood volume = 80 ml/kg.
One gram of Hb contains 3.4 mg iron.
The factor 1.5 is used to provide the extra iron to replace body stores.

PREPARATIONS

Iron dextran complex (Imferon) 2 ml and 5 ml preparations contain 50 mg of elemental iron/ml. Iron-sorbitol citric acid complex (Jectofer) 2 ml ampoules contain 50 mg elemental iron/ml.

RESPONSE RATE

Oral and parenteral iron cause a response at about the same time. Reticulocyte levels peak between the fifth and tenth day. A rise in haemoglobin begins at about one week, after the peak reticulocyte response. The haemoglobin can be expected to rise by 2 g/dl every 3 weeks.

CAUSES OF A FAILURE TO RESPOND TO IRON THERAPY

1 Failure to give the iron.
2 Inadequate dosage or ineffective preparation.
3 Impaired absorption.
4 Continued blood loss.
5 Incorrect diagnosis.
6 Coexisting disease (e.g. renal failure).
7 Coexisting folate deficiency.
8 Sideroblastic anaemia.

Rare causes of microcytic hypochromic anaemia

Congenital atransferrinaemia A rare autosomal recessive condition which gives rise to a severe hypochromic microcytic anaemia present at birth. There is an unexplained haemosiderosis in spite of the almost complete absence of the plasma iron transport protein. The disease responds to intravenous transferrin.

Defective iron mobilization with IgA deficiency

A condition resembling idiopathic pulmonary haemosiderosis. Iron is lost into the lungs because of a defect in the macrophage system. There is a low serum iron and poor iron reutilization. The anaemia responds to iron therapy. An IgA deficiency is an associated feature.

Sideroblastic anaemia

A rare condition in childhood which is characterized by the presence of ring sideroblasts (stainable iron in clumps around the nucleus) in the bone marrow. The causes of sideroblastic anaemia are due to a variety of enzyme abnormalities, either primary or secondary, as seen in association with lead poisoning and rare dietary deficiencies of pyridoxine. In patients who clearly have neither lead poisoning nor dietary pyridoxine deficiency, large doses of pyridoxine may give a complete or partial response, but the patients are pyridoxine dependent.

RECOMMENDED READING

Bothwell T.H. & Finch C.A. (1979) *Iron Metabolism.* Blackwell Scientific Publications, Oxford.

Burman D. (1972) Haemoglobin levels in normal infants aged 3 to 24 months and the effect of iron. *Archives of the Diseases of Childhood* **47**, 261.

Charlton R.W. & Bothwell T.H. (1970) Iron deficiency anemia. *Seminars in Hematology* 7, 67.

Committee on Nutrition (1969) Iron balance and requirements in infancy. *Pediatrics* **43**, 134.

Dallman P.R. (1974) Iron, vitamin E, and folate in the preterm infant. *Journal of Pediatrics* **85**, 742.

Dallman P.R. (1974) The nutritional anemias. In *Hematology of Infancy and Childhood* (eds D.G. Nathan & F.A. Oski). W.B. Saunders, Philadelphia.

Harris J.W. & Kellermeyer R.W. (1970) Iron lack anemia. In *The Red Cell. Production, Metabolism and Destruction: normal and abnormal*, 2nd edn, p.64. Harvard University Press, Mass.

Jacobs A. (1974) Erythropoiesis and iron-deficiency anaemia. *Iron in Biochemistry and Medicine* (eds A. Jacobs & M. Worwood), p.405. Academic Press, London.

Lanzkowsky P. (1961) The influence of maternal iron-deficiency anaemia on the haemoglobin of the infant. *Archives of the Diseases of Childhood* **36**, 205.

Lovric V.A., Lammi A.T. & Friend J.C.M. (1972) Nutrition, iron intake and haematological status in healthy children. *Medical Journal of Australia* **I**, 11.

Siimes M.A., Addiego J.I. & Dallman P.R. (1974) Ferritin in serum: diagnosis of iron deficiency and iron overload in infants and children. *Blood* **43**, 581.

Turnbull A. (1974) Iron absorption. In *Iron in Biochemistry and Medicine* (eds A. Jacobs & M. Worwood), p.369. Academic Press, London.

Wallerstein R.O. (1968) Intravenous iron-dextran complex. *Blood* **32**, 690.

Chapter 10
Megaloblastic Anaemias

General characteristics and causes

In children, dietary folic acid deficiency is the commonest cause of megaloblastic anaemia and is often associated with iron deficiency. Vitamin B_{12} deficiency is a rare cause of megaloblastic anaemia, but may occur as either a nutritional disorder, as a malabsorption due to lack of production of intrinsic factor or a specific malabsorption. The remaining causes are very rare and are listed in Table 10.1.

Clinical features

Folate deficiency may occur at any age from 4 months. Vitamin B_{12} deficiency due to congenital malabsorption is detected in the first 3 years of life, while early onset pernicious anaemia may occur from 8 years of age.

The onset of symptoms is insidious. Pallor, weight loss, apathy, anorexia, diarrhoea and regression of mile stones may occur. The skin is a 'lemon yellow' colour due to mild jaundice in addition to the skin pallor. The tongue may be sore, red and show a loss of papillae. Parasthesia and neuropathy may

Table 10.1 Causes of megaloblastic anaemias.

Folate deficiency
Vitamin B_{12} deficiency
Childhood pernicious anaemia
Childhood pernicious anaemia associated with endocrine abnormalities
Small bowel disorders
Selective malabsorption
Defect of Vitamin B_{12} transport proteins
Miscellaneous
Orotic aciduria
Congenital enzyme abnormalities involving formation of folate coenzymes
Drug induced megaloblastosis due to interference with purine pyrimidine production or ribonucleatide reductase activity
Acquired defects of DNA synthesis (e.g. sideroblastic anaemia, leukaemia, aplastic anaemia, liver disease).

rarely occur with vitamin B_{12} deficiency. Subacute combined degeneration of the cord may occur in patients with vitamin B_{12} deficiency who have had the diagnosis delayed. Neuropathy does not appear to occur with folate deficiency. Moderate splenomegaly occurs in about half of the patients. Bruising may occur in severe megaloblastosis due to thrombocytopenia.

Laboratory investigations

BLOOD EXAMINATION

Anaemia, sometimes severe, is present. The red cells show an oval macrocytosis, accompanied by anisocytosis and poikilocytosis. Associated iron deficiency may mask the red cell changes of megaloblastic anaemia. There may be a moderate neutropenia, the neutrophils showing increased lobe segmentation. Mild to severe thrombocytopenia may occur.

BONE MARROW EXAMINATION

Bone marrow changes occur in the developing erythroblasts, granulocytes and megakaryocytes being most obvious in the late erythroblasts. The erythroblasts are large, the nucleus shows poor chromatin condensation and there is a relative dissociation of maturation of the nucleus compared to the haemoglobinization of the cytoplasm. Cytoplasmic stippling is present and Howell-Jolly bodies are prominent. Mitoses are more common than normal. Chromosome preparations show the chromatids to be large and breaks are common. The developing granulocytes are large, with greatly enlarged nuclei, particularly in the metamyelocytes and band forms. Megakaryocytes may show agranular cytoplasm or be hypersegmented. Iron stores are increased when the marrow is stained with potassium ferrocyanide. The erythroblasts show fine iron staining granules throughout the cytoplasm.

Coexistent iron deficiency masks the red cell changes, erythropoiesis being micronormoblastic. Diagnosis is possible by observing the megaloblastic changes in granulopoiesis, which are not masked by the presence of iron deficiency.

A large element of intra-marrow death of the red cells and leucocytes is present, giving rise to mild jaundice. Red cell survival is decreased, with an increase of unconjugated bilirubin in the plasma.

Diagnosis

The diagnosis is made by examination of the blood and bone marrow aspiration films. Levels of folic acid in the serum and red cells are assayed microbiologically using *Lactobacillus casei*, or by use of the radioimmunoassay. The level of vitamin B_{12} in the serum is assayed microbiologically using *Euglena gracilis*, *Lactobacillus leishmanni* or *Ochromonas malhamenis*.

Isotope dilution techniques are available for assay of vitamin B_{12}. The estimation of the serum levels of both folic acid and vitamin B_{12} should be carried out in all patients.

Further tests may be appropriate, mainly applying to patients with vitamin B_{12} deficiency: Absorption tests of vitamin B_{12}, without and with added intrinsic factor (Schilling test); determination of antibodies directed against intrinsic factor, parietal cells, thryoid, reticulin and immunoglobulins; tests for gastric atrophy, presence of gastric acid, intestinal malabsorption.

FOLATE DEFICIENCY

REQUIREMENTS

The minimum daily requirement of folate is thought to be 25–50 ng in infants, 50–75 ng in adults. Total body stores vary from 6–20 mg, so that there is only sufficient supply for a few months. Megaloblastic anaemia can develop after 4 months on a folate-free diet.

Normal dietary intake is around 0.2–0.5 mg. Foods with the highest folate content are yeast, liver, kidney, nuts, leafy green vegetables and citrus fruit. Cows milk is a poor source of folate (35 ng/l). Heating of foods, especially in large volumes of water, may destroy up to 95% of the folates.

ABSORPTION AND TRANSPORT

Absorption occurs in the duodenum and jejunum. About 50% of natural folates are absorbed. They enter the portal blood as 5-methyltetrahydrofolate following deconjugation, reduction and methylation, either in the intestine or in the luminal cell. Synthetic folic acid is absorbed more readily than natural folate. Absorption is probably by saturation, although an active absorption mechanism probably exists.

No plasma transport protein is known. Normal plasma levels vary between 3 and 20 ng/ml. The fetus absorbs folate preferentially from the maternal circulation, so that the cord folate level is twice the maternal level. There is a period of marginal folate balance until about one year after birth, when normal adult levels are attained. Premature infants are at greater risk of folate deficiency in the period 1–3 months than infants of normal birth weight.

ROLE IN CELL METABOLISM

Folic acid is reduced by dihydrofolate reductase to form tetrahydrofolic acid. A number of tetra hydrofolate coenzymes are subsequently formed which are involved in the transfer of carbon units from one compound to another. Probably the most important reaction in which a folate coenzyme is involved, is the methylation of deoxyuridylate to thymidylate, a rate-limiting step in the synthesis of DNA. The enzyme dihydrofolate reductase occupies a critical position in reduction of folic acid to its tetrahydro coenzymes. The affinity of the cytotoxic agent, methotrexate, for this enzyme is greater than that of folic acid, and by inhibiting the activity of dihydrofolate reductase, methotrexate interferes with DNA synthesis. Other reactions involved include purine synthesis and amino acid interconversion, which are listed in Table 10.2.

Causes of folate deficiency

NUTRITION

Nutritional folate deficiency is the commonest cause of megaloblastic anaemia. This is especially so in the first year after birth, when the low content of cow's milk (35 ng/l) may be decreased by up to 40% by heating. Children fed with goat's milk (6 ng/l) are especially vulnerable to folate deficiency. Dietary lack of folate usually results from overcooking the food rather than lack of provision of folate containing foods. Folate deficiency is often associated with protein-calorie malnutrition, scurvy and iron deficiency. Occasionally, a dietary lack of vitamin B_{12} may occur with folate deficiency.

MALABSORPTION

Coeliac disease, idiopathic steatorrhoea and tropical sprue are often accompanied by folate deficiency. The mechanism of production is probably

Table 10.2 Reactions involved in folate deficiency.

Reaction	Co-enzyme involved (THF = Tetrahydrofolate)	Carbon unit transferred
Pyrimidine synthesis: deoxyuridine to thymidine	5,10-methenyl THF	$-CH_3$
Purine synthesis: formylation of glycine amide ribotide	5,10-methenyl THF	-CH0
Formylation of aicar	10-formyl THF	-CH0
Formate activation of THF	THF	-CH0
Amino acid Homocysteine to methionine	5-methyl THF	$-CH_3$
Serine to glycine	THF	$-CH_2$
Formiminoglutamic acid to glutamic acid	THF	-CH=NH-

multifactorial, and includes loss of intestinal conjugase activity, a loss of the intestinal flora leading to a decrease in production of folate and possibly a decrease in absorption due to excessively rapid intestinal passage.

Extensive jejunal resection, partial resection of the stomach and Crohn's disease usually cause folate deficiency due to poor nutrition. Drugs (phenytoin, oral contraceptives) appear to cause folate deficiency because of their ability to inhibit the activity of the intestinal conjugases.

Rare congenital cases of selective malabsorption have been described.

INCREASED UTILIZATION

Increased amounts of folate are required in premature infants, haematological disorders with high output states (haemolytic anaemias, thalassaemia, sickle cell disease, hereditary spherocytosis), malignancies (acute leukaemia), chronic inflammatory diseases (tuberculosis, bacterial endocarditis, etc.) and following long-term dialysis.

ANTIFOLATE DRUGS

Drugs given in the treatment of neoplasma, e.g. methotrexate, aminopterin and the drug trimethoprim exert an inhibitory effect on the enzyme dihydrofolate reductase (see Chapter 7).

Other drugs involved in the occurrence of folate associated megaloblastosis are the anticonvulsants, phenytoin and primidone, and alcohol.

CONGENITAL DISORDERS

A small number of patients have been described with enzyme abnormalities, resulting in megaloblastic anaemia of folate deficiency. These include dihydrofolate reductase, N^5 methyltetrahydrofolate homocysteine methyltransferase deficiency and some patients with formimino-transferase deficiency.

Treatment

Folic acid tablets 1–5 mg/day should be given until anaemia is corrected. Reticulocytosis can be expected 2–3 days after commencing treatment. A rise in Hb levels occurs after one week of treatment.

In severely ill children where urgent treatment is required, folic acid and vitamin B_{12} should be administered parenterally and a slow packed red cell transfusion, aimed at elevating the haemoglobin level by 3 g%, should be given. Vitamin B_{12} is administered to ensure that folic acid does not precipitate the appearance of subacute combined degeneration of the cord, which can occur in children with true vitamin B_{12} deficiency.

Folate and iron deficiency often coexist. Response to treatment with folic acid may be limited by the iron deficiency. When there is a dietary cause of folate deficiency, both folate and iron should be administered to obtain optimum response.

VITAMIN B_{12}

NATURAL SOURCES AND REQUIREMENTS

A number of chemical forms of vitamin B_{12} exist. It was first isolated as the compound, cyanocobalamin. The only source of vitamin B_{12} for man is animal protein food. Heart, liver and kidney are the best sources, with muscle meat, chicken, fish, eggs, cheese and milk containing lesser amounts. Vegetables contain virtually no vitamin B_{12}.

Daily needs are about 1–3 μg, normal diets supply 3–30 μg. Body stores are about 3–5 mg, enough for 2–4 years' supply.

ABSORPTION AND TRANSPORT

Absorption is both passive and active. Passive absorption occurs throughout the jejunum and ileum, but is less than 1% of ingested vitamin B_{12}. Active absorption is the most important. Food vitamin B_{12} is released from its protein by the action of gastric acid and proteolytic enzymes and combines with a glycoprotein of molecular weight 60 000, intrinsic factor, secreted by the gastric parietal cells. The intrinsic factor — Vitamin B_{12} complex binds to receptor sites on the mucosal cells of the terminal ileum, where the vitamin B_{12} is absorbed. The mechanism involved in the absorption of vitamin B_{12} is not known.

Transport of vitamin B_{12} to the liver and other minor store areas (heart, brain and kidneys) is accomplished by two major proteins, transcobalamin I (TC I) and transcobalamin II (TC II). TC I is an α_1-globulin (MW 60 000) which is probably made by granulocytes and carries 90% of the circulating Vitamin B_{12}. TC II is a β-globulin (MW 38 000) and carries little of the circulating vitamin B_{12}. It is essential for the passage of vitamin B_{12} in and out of cells and for transport between organs.

ROLE IN CELL METABOLISM

Vitamin B_{12} appears to take part in only two reactions in man. The first involves the isomerization of methymalonyl-CoA to succinyl-CoA, using deoxyadenosylcobalamin. The second reaction, the methylation of homocysteine to methionine, involves methyl B_{12} and methyltetrahydrofolic acid. It is thought that deficiency of vitamin B_{12} traps methyltetrahydrofolate at this step, causing the reduced folate coenzyme to be unavailable for DNA synthesis. This hypothesis is termed the 'methylfolate trap' theory.

Causes of vitamin B_{12} deficiency

NUTRITIONAL

This is very rare in most communities. Children breast fed for long periods by vitamin B_{12} deficient mothers may develop megaloblastic anaemia in the first two years of life. Children given a strictly vegetarian diet may become megaloblastic.

DEFECTIVE ABSORPTION

Absence of intrinsic factor may cause congenital pernicious anaemia, with megaloblastic anaemia occurring before the age of 3 years. No other congenital abnormalities are present. Inheritance is autosomal recessive.

Disorders of vitamin B_{12} metabolism

JUVENILE PERNICIOUS ANAEMIA

This is an autoimmune disease resembling adult pernicious anaemia, but occurring about the age of 8 years. Gastric atrophy, absent intrinsic factor, a high incidence of antibody to intrinsic factor and low incidence of parietal cell antibody are present. A small proportion of these patients have been described with an associated IgA deficiency. Therapy with vitamin B_{12} resolved the anaemia, but the IgA deficiency remained.

JUVENILE PERNICIOUS ANAEMIA WITH ENDOCRINOPATHIES

This disorder resembles adult pernicious anaemia, but with associated various endocrinopathies (hypoparathyroidism, Addison's disease, myxoedema).

SMALL INTESTINE MALABSORPTION

More than 80 patients have been described with a familial disorder of absorption of vitamin B_{12} in the ileum. Megaloblastic anaemia occurs before 3 years of age, usually associated with a benign proteinuria without renal disease in most patients. The anaemia responds to parenteral vitamin B_{12}, but the proteinuria remains.

GENERAL MALABSORPTION

Small bowel disease may result in a megaloblastic anaemia due to vitamin B_{12} malabsorption. Crohn's disease, bowel resection, chronic diarrhoea and malignancies of the bowel may all be associated with megaloblastosis.

INTESTINAL INFECTION

Bacterial overgrowth, occurring in the blind loop syndrome, and diverticulosis appear to be responsible for Vitamin B_{12} deficiency because of the utilization of the Vitamin B_{12} by the bacteria. Infestation with the fish tape worm, diphyllobothrium latum, appears to cause Vitamin B_{12} deficiency by the same mechanism.

DEFECTIVE TRANSPORT

Congenital deficiency of the transport protein, transcobalamin II, is an uncommon cause of severe megaloblastosis presenting in the early weeks after birth. Treatment is with massive doses of Vitamin B_{12}.

CONGENITAL DISORDERS OF VITAMIN B_{12} METABOLISM

A number of patients have been shown to have an inability to form the Vitamin B_{12} coenzyme, adenosylcobalamin. The marked ketoacidosis, often accompanied by hypoglycaemia, may result in early death. Megaloblastosis is not associated with this disorder.

Abnormalities of formation of methylcobalamin and adrenylcobalamin has been described in a few patients. Two were seriously affected, had megaloblastic anaemia, and died aged 7 weeks and 7 years. Two less seriously affected patients failed to show megaloblastosis.

Treatment

Vitamin B_{12} deficiency responds to physiological doses (1 μg) of hydroxycobalamin given over a 10 day period. The usual doses in children are 200–1000 μg given by intramuscular injection every month for life. Transcobalamin II deficiency only responds to massive doses of vitamin B_{12} (1000 μg every 2–3 days).

If the anaemia is severe and treatment is urgent, both vitamin B_{12} and folate should be given. Folate should not be given alone, as it may precipitate subacute combined degeneration of the cord in vitamin B_{12} induced megaloblastic anaemia.

RECOMMENDED READING

Chanarin I. (1979) *The Megaloblastic Anaemias*, 2nd edn. Blackwell Scientific Publications, Oxford.

Erbe R.W. (1975) Inborn errors of folate metabolism. *New England Journal of Medicine* **293**, 753.

Furuhjelm U. & Nevanlinna H.R. (1973) Inheritance of selective malabsorption of vitamin B_{12}. *Scandinavian Journal of Haematology* **II**, 27.

HAKAMI N., NEIMAN P.E., CANELLOS G.P. *et al.* (1971) Neonatal megaloblastic anemia due to inherited transcobalamin II deficiency in 2 siblings. *New England Journal of Medicine* **285**, 1163.

HARRIS J.W. & KELLERMEYER R.W. (1970) *The Red Cell. Production, metabolism, destruction: normal and abnormal*, 2nd edn, p.334. Harvard University Press, Cambridge, Mass.

HERBERT V. (ed.) (1970) Symposium on vitamin B_{12} and folate. *American Journal of Medicine* **48**, 539.

HERBERT V. (1975) Drugs effective in megaloblastic anemias. Vitamin B_{12} and folic acid. In *The Pharmacological Basis of Therapeutics* (eds L.S. Goodman & A. Gilman), 5th edn. Macmillan, New York.

HOFFBRAND A.V. (1971) The megaloblastic anaemias. In *Recent Advances in Haematology* (eds A. Goldberg & M.C. Brain). Churchill Livingstone, Edinburgh.

HOFFBRAND A.V. (1970) Folate deficiency in premature infants. *Archives of Diseases of Childhood* **45**, 441.

IMERSLUND O. & PAL B. (1963) Familial vitamin B_{12} malabsorption. *Acta Haematologica* **30**, 1.

LANCET EDITORIAL (1973) Folate deficiency in childhood. *Lancet* **1**, 813.

MCINTYRE O.R., SULLIVAN L.W., JEFFRIES G.H. *et al.* (1965) Pernicious anemia in childhood. *New England Journal of Medicine* **272**, 981.

MAHONEY M.J. & ROSENBERG L.E. (1970) Inherited defects of B_{12} metabolism. *American Journal of Medicine* **48**, 584.

MILLER D.R., BLOOM G.E., STREIFF R.R. *et al.* (1966) Juvenile 'congenital' pernicious anemia. *New England Journal of Medicine* **275**, 978.

STEBBINS R., SCOTT J. & HERBERT V. (1973) Drug-induced megaloblastic anemias. *Seminars in Hematology* **10**, 235.

STREIFF R.R. (1970) Folic acid deficiency anemia. *Seminars in Hematology* **7**, 23.

Chapter 11
Aplastic Anaemias; Congenital Dyserythropoietic Anaemia and Osteopetrosis

Bone marrow failure in infants and children is an uncommon, but important, group of disorders.

Bone marrow failure may be either absolute or relative to increased demands on haematopoiesis, as is seen with the aplastic crises of haemolytic anaemias and some haemoglobinopathies. Absolute failure is seen in congenital and acquired aplastic anaemias, including Fanconi's anaemia and pure red cell aplasia.

CONGENITAL PURE RED CELL APLASIA (Diamond-Blackfan syndrome)

This disease is the result of complete or almost complete failure of bone marrow erythropoiesis. There is normal granulocyte and platelet production. It must be distinguished from acquired pure red cell aplasia which is more common in adults, the secondary red cell aplasias associated with toxins, drugs, autoimmune diseases, some viral infections and aplastic crises occurring with hereditary haemolytic anaemias.

Aetiology

The cause is uncertain, but is currently thought to be due to a failure of the erythropoietic stem cell to respond to the differentiating influence of erythropoietin. Lymphocyte induced inhibitors of erythroid colony formation have recently been described, but their role in the aetiology of congenital pure red cell aplasia is unknown.

Both autosomal recessive and autosomal dominant inheritance have been described.

Clinical features

Anaemia usually presents within the first year of life. A proportion (15%) are evident at birth while, in some, the onset may be delayed until as late as 6 years of age. A characteristic facies is described, with wide set eyes, thick lips, snub nose and an intelligent expression. Congenital abnormalities are described in about one-quarter of the patients, including skeletal abnormalities involving the radial side of the arm, webbed neck, cardiac abnormalities, cleft lip and palate, malformed ears, growth and mental retardation and minor chromosomal abnormalities.

The anaemia is normocytic, normochromic. Reticulocytes are absent from the peripheral blood. Other elements of the peripheral blood are normal. Bone marrow examination reveals absent or near absent erythropoiesis, other elements being normal. If erythroblasts are seen, they are the earliest recognizable cells, the pronormoblasts. Haemosiderosis may be present late in the disease.

Differential diagnosis

Aplastic anaemia is distinguished by the reduction or absence of all other marrow elements. Temporary red cell hypoplasia which may follow erythroblastosis fetalis may be confused with pure red cell aplasia. An acute red cell aplasia may also occur secondary to a variety of toxic events (see Acquired Red Cell Aplasia) and may be difficult to differentiate from the Diamond-Blackfan syndrome. The relatively rapid recovery of secondary pure red cell aplasia is the main distinguishing feature.

Treatment

Corticosteroids produce a response in almost all patients if commenced within 3 months of diagnosis. Delay in starting treatment beyond 3 months reduces the response rate, two-thirds responding if treatment begins before 12 months, while no response is seen if treatment is delayed for 3 years. Prednisone given in a dose of 2 mg/kg/day in three divided doses will usually cause a response in 1–3 weeks. The dose is then reduced to the minimum maintenance dose required to maintain a normal haemoglobin level. Failure to respond after a 2 month trial of steroids should lead to discontinuation of this treatment. Androgenic steroids have no proven value in this disorder.

Transfusion may be required to support patients who do not respond to prednisone. Complications due to development of leucocyte or platelet antibodies may be avoided by use of frozen and thawed red cells. Haemosiderosis will eventually follow any transfusion regimen. Prevention of transfusion haemosiderosis is described in Chapter 13. Splenectomy may be necessary if hypersplenism occurs, but is not recommended otherwise.

Prognosis

Spontaneous recovery occurs in about one-third of the patients, while steroids cause remission in about one-half. The prognosis of the remainder is guarded, death being due to haemosiderosis or due to infection. Several children with this disorder have developed acute non-lymphocytic leukaemia in early adult life.

ACUTE TRANSIENT RED CELL APLASIA

This condition may occur as a complication of blood disorders which impose long-standing haematopoietic stress, or as a direct toxic effect on bone marrow function. It is responsible for the aplastic crises seen in congenital haemolytic anaemias (e.g. hereditary spherocytosis), chronic autoimmune haemolytic anaemias or be secondary to viral infections, bacterial sepsis and drug exposure. Lists of drugs which have been reported to be associated with transient anaemia can be obtained from undesirable drug effects registers.

The characteristic clinical feature of this condition is the appearance of unexpected anaemia. Blood examination shows normocytic, normochromic anaemia with reticulocytopenia. Bone marrow examination reveals decreased erythropoiesis. Recovery of bone marrow function is usually rapid and is often in progress by the time the condition is clinically apparent. Severe anaemia is treated by transfusion. There is no evidence that corticosteroids accelerate recovery.

ACQUIRED RED CELL APLASIA

In adults and adolescents, pure red cell aplasia may develop in association with autoimmune disorders and/or a thymoma. The presence of an IgG inhibitor of erythropoiesis, with either an elevated erythropoietin level or an absence or near absence of erythropoietin, has been demonstrated in some of these patients. In other patients, there is absence of the inhibitor and erythropoietin. In patients with thymoma, thymectomy results in a cure in about 25%. Immunosuppression therapy using cyclophosphamide has been successful in patients with documented IgG inhibitors of erythropoiesis.

APLASTIC ANAEMIAS

Aplastic anaemia follows the failure of the bone marrow to produce red cells, leucocytes or platelets. This pancytopenia is due to either a depletion of the stem cells or interference with their capacity to produce the cells capable of maturation into the various lines of haemopoietic cells.

Classification

1 Acquired aplastic anaemia.
(a) Idiopathic.

(b) Secondary to exposure to drugs, chemicals, infectious hepatitis, infections (e.g. tuberculosis, infectious mononucleosis), in association with pancreatic insufficiency, associated with paroxymal nocturnal haemoglobinuria.
2 Constitutional aplastic anaemia.
(a) With congenital abnormalities (Fanconi's anaemia).
(b) Without congenital abnormalities.

ACQUIRED APLASTIC ANAEMIA

While this disorder is relatively rare (3.5–5.4 cases/million population), it is important because of the severity, morbidity and mortality which ensue.

Aetiology

No cause can be determined in at least one-half of the patients. Drugs, chemicals or infections are incriminated in the remainder.

DRUGS

The list of drugs associated with marrow depression is large and the reader is referred to undesirable drug effects registers. A small number of drugs will be detailed because of frequent or particular association with marrow depression.

Antineoplastic drugs invariably cause marrow depression to some degree. The degree of depression varies with the drug or drug combination and is almost invariably recoverable on withdrawal of the drug. Large doses of some of the drugs (cyclophosphamide) are used prior to marrow transplantation to ablate the marrow and immune system.

Chloramphenicol causes aplastic anaemia in approximately 1/30 000 users. Two types of aplasia occur. The first is an idiosyncratic reaction and is probably irreversible. The second appears to be dose related and of a toxic nature, from which recovery occurs following withdrawal of the drug.

Phenylbutazone and oxyphenylbutazone only rarely cause aplasia in children, probably because of their infrequent use. Overall, they are the commonest causes of aplastic anaemia. The risk is around 1 in 24 000. The aplasia usually follows prolonged use of the drug and is often severe.

CHEMICALS

Benzene is a highly volatile, aromatic hydrocarbon produced from coal tar, widely used as organic solvents. Aplasia may be induced by inhalation or ingestion and is frequently severe.

The time interval may be either short or years after exposure. The marrow aplasia may be succeeded by the development of acute leukaemia, usually non-lymphoid. Aplasia has been described following glue sniffing and the use of synthetic hair dyes.

INFECTIONS

Infectious hepatitis Aplastic anaemia following infectious hepatitis is rare, but has an ominous outlook, with a very high mortality rate. There is a slight male predominance (60%). The hepatitis itself is usually not severe. A small number of cases of aplastic anaemia have been associated with infectious mononucleosis.

An association with paroxymal nocturnal haemoglobinuria is also described.

Clinical features

The onset is gradual, with bleeding manifestations as the most common presenting feature. Pallor and fatigue are also frequently present. Symptoms of infections are less common at initial presentation, but become marked with progress of the disease. The liver and spleen are not enlarged, and there is no lymphadenopathy.

Laboratory investigations

Investigations reveal moderate to marked normocytic, normochromic anaemia with reticulocytopenia, leucopenia with a profound neutropenia and marked thrombocytopenia. Bone marrow aspirations at a number of sites, together with marrow trephine, reveal marrow hypocellularity, with a marked reduction of all the cellular components. Occasionally, a progressive fall in all blood and bone marrow components may be seen over a number of weeks or months. Local areas of normocellular marrow may be found but, overall, marrow failure is the predominant feature. Occasionally, acute leukaemia can present with an aplastic phase which usually responds rapidly to corticosteroid therapy but, subsequently, frank leukaemia becomes apparent.

Prognostic features

Reviews of survival curves in non-transplanted patients suggest that there are two broad categories of patients; one with a mortality rate of more than 90%, the other with a long-term survival of 50–70%.

The following have been shown to be associated with poor prognosis:

1 Haemorrhagic onset of the disease.
2 Male sex.
3 Short interval from first symptoms to hospitalization.
4 Mean reticulocyte count $< 1\%$.

5 Neutrophil count $< 0.5 \times 10^9/l$.
6 Platelet count $< 20 \times 10^9/l$.
7 Marked marrow hypocellularity with non-myeloid cells > 70%.

Treatment

It is now well established that the treatment of choice in patients with poor prognostic features is bone marrow transplantation, which has at least a 50% cure rate. The highest success rate with this procedure is obtained in patients in whom transfusions have been avoided and who have HLA compatible siblings. Therefore, at presentation, it is essential to perform red cell and HLA grouping and mixed lymphocyte cultures on the patient and the siblings. If transfusion therapy is required as a life-saving procedure, red cells should be given in the form of frozen red cells, while platelet and granulocyte transfusions should be given from one or two unrelated donors. Infections should be treated with appropriate intravenous antibiotics of broad spectrum type. There is no objective evidence that androgen therapy is of any benefit in these patients and such treatment should be avoided if there is any possibility of transplantation. In patients with a HLA and mixed lymphocyte culture compatible sibling, informed consent for bone marrow transplantation should be obtained from the donor and parents.

Transplantation is most successful in centres with experience in this procedure. The details of bone marrow transplantation and management of graft versus host disease are beyond the scope of this book, but are well described in the literature (Thomas *et al.* 1975. *New England Journal of Medicine* **292**, 832.).

In patients without features of poor prognosis, there is a high spontaneous remission rate. As there are considerable risks to the procedure of bone marrow transplantation and the complications of graft versus host disease, in the majority of such patients conservative treatment should be tried. There is anecdotal experience that recovery can be accelerated with the use of androgens (oxymethalone 2–5 mg/kg), but randomized studies show no significant difference between groups of patients treated with or without androgens. Spontaneous or androgen induced remissions are slow and incomplete. The majority of patients have residual thrombocytopenia and neutropenia. These can be clinically significant if the patients become infected. Amongst patients without features of poor prognosis, there are some who will deteriorate and develop features of poor prognosis. If possible, such patients should be promptly transplanted.

In patients with poor prognosis, but no compatible marrow donors, it may be of value to attempt therapy with antithymocyte globulin or immuno-suppressive therapy such as cyclophosphamide, as there are reports in the literature of occasional responses to this form of treatment. New developments in overcoming transplantation graft versus host reactions may become applicable to this group of patients in the future but, until then, their prognosis remains very poor.

CONSTITUTIONAL APLASTIC ANAEMIAS

A number of congenital aplastic anaemias have been described:
1 Fanconi's anaemia. Progressive congenital pancytopenia associated with chromosomal abnormalities and congenital skin, renal, nervous system and skeletal anomalies.
2 Constitutional aplastic anaemia. Progressive pancytopenia without congenital abnormalities.
3 Dyskeratosis congenita. Pancytopenia with increased skin pigmentation, mental retardation and decreased growth. Oesophageal diverticula, teeth dysplasia and skin telangiectasia may be present. No chromosome, renal or skeletal abnormalities are present.

Fanconi's anaemia

CLINICAL FEATURES

The abnormalities associated with Fanconi's anaemia are present at birth. They include hyperpigmentation of the skin of the central part of the body, present in three-quarters of the patients; short stature due to a shortened trunk; renal abnormalities (absent kidney, horseshoe kidney, hydronephrosis); and skeletal abnormalities which most often involve the upper limbs (absent thumbs, absent or hypoplastic first metacarpal, decreased wrist ossification centres, triphalangeal thumbs, hypoplasia of the thumb nail). The radius may be absent from one or both forearms. Many other skeletal abnormalities are described. The central nervous system may be affected, with mental retardation, microphthalmia, microcephaly, deafness, external auditory canal stenosis, strabismus, nystagmus and hyper-reflexia.

The pancytopenia may commence as early as 17 months, but may be delayed until the third decade. The mean age for presentation is 6.6 years for boys and 8.8 years for girls. Thrombocytopenia usually develops first, followed by neutropenia and anaemia over a period of months to several years. The inheritance is uncertain, some evidence favouring a recessive inheritance with variable penetrance, other indicating dominant inheritance. There is a high incidence of leukaemic transformation in these patients.

INVESTIGATIONS

The bone marrow may show megaloblastic erythroid hyperplasia at first, but is eventually replaced by a hypoplastic marrow. Chromosome examination of fibroblasts and transformed lymphocytes shows breaks, gaps, constrictions and translocations. Skeletal survey and intravenous pyelogram demonstrate congenital abnormalities.

TREATMENT

Most patients respond to androgens. A wide range of androgens have been used, but there is no evidence that one preparation is superior to another. Oxymethalone 2–5 mg/kg/day is usually well tolerated. Response to androgens is slow. Initially, there is a rise in reticulocyte count followed by a rise in the haemoglobin. There is partial improvement of the neutrophil count but little, if any, effect of androgens on the platelet count.

The duration of androgen treatment is controversial because of its masculinizing effects, further impairment of growth in children who, in any case, are growing poorly and the risk of developing hepatic adenomas or carcinoma. There is also some suggestion that long-term androgen treatment may accelerate conversion to leukaemia. For these reasons, androgens should be gradually withdrawn once a response has been obtained. If possible, the patients should be maintained without androgens. If anaemia recurs, then the minimum dose of androgens should be used. It is wise to check on α-fetoprotein levels during the course of androgen treatment. If these become elevated, a liver scan should be performed, looking for a hepatic adenoma, and androgen therapy discontinued. A failure to respond to a 4 month course of androgen indicates that further trials of androgen therapy are not warranted.

As in acquired aplastic anaemia, bone marrow transplantation may offer a cure of the aplastic anaemia. Transfusion of blood products should therefore be avoided. If this is not possible, frozen red cells and granulocytes and platelets from unrelated donors should be used. Donor compatibility of siblings should be ascertained, as discussed in the section on acquired aplastic anaemia. For reasons which are not understood, bone marrow transplantation is less successful in Fanconi's anaemia than in idiopathic aplastic anaemia. Rejection of the graft appears to be a particular problem.

Constitutional aplastic anaemia

CLINICAL FEATURES AND DIAGNOSIS

This condition is more common than Fanconi's anaemia. It usually presents as a progressive pancytopenia in children with short stature, but no other congenital abnormalities. Thrombocytopenia is the earliest presenting feature and, in the early stages of the disease, this condition may be confused with chronic ITP. The diagnosis is confirmed by bone marrow aspiration and trephine.

TREATMENT

There is often a partial response to androgens, as described in the section on Fanconi's anaemia. There is no evidence that there is a high frequency of leukaemic conversion.

Congenital dyserythropoietic anaemia (CDA)

This rare group of disorders is characterized by ineffective erythropoiesis, erythroblast multinuclearity and haemosiderosis. Four types are described, but there is overlap between each type and variation within type. The patients often present with mild anaemia. Hepatosplenomegaly is often present. There may be episodes of jaundice associated with haemolysis and more severe anaemia. Development of gallstones and haemosiderosis are late complications of the disorder. There is no specific treatment — transfusion is required if the anaemia is severe.

CLASSIFICATION

Type I Reported from birth to 32 years, showing peripheral blood macrocytosis. Bone marrow erythroblasts show intranuclear bridges and have megaloblastoid morphology. Electron microscopic changes are non-specific. Inheritance is autosomal recessive. About one-sixth of the patients with CDA are Type I.

Type II Occurring from birth to 30 years, the peripheral blood shows anisocytosis, poikilocytosis and polychromasia. The marrow erythroblasts show binuclear and multinuclear changes and, on electron microscopy, show a double cytoplasmic membrane. The acid serum test (Ham's test) is positive with two-thirds of the sera tested, and antibodies directed against the *I* antigen and *i* antigen are found. Inheritance is autosomal recessive. About two-thirds of the reported patients are of this type.

Type III Reported from 2 months to the seventh decade, the peripheral blood shows macrocytosis. The bone marrow erythroblasts are huge, showing up to 12 nuclei. Electron microscopic changes are non-specific. There is autosomal dominant inheritance. About one-sixth of the patients are of this type.

Type IV Occurs in about 5% of patients. It has been reported in patients aged 19 months to 51 years. Multinuclearity is present in about one-third of the marrow erythroblasts and resembles that seen in Type II, but there are serological abnormalities.

OSTEOPETROSIS

Osteopetrosis is characterized by an overgrowth of osseous material in the bone marrow, causing marrow failure by replacement. The condition may be present from birth, but may be delayed for a number of decades. There is progressive haemopoietic failure, characterized by anaemia, thrombocytopenia and transient leucocytosis which progresses to leucopenia. The red cells show the characteristic tear-drop shape seen in marrow replacement. The bones are hard and brittle, with spontaneous and easily induced fractures which heal poorly. X-rays show a replacement of the marrow cavity with cortical bone. Neurological signs include facial paralysis and optic atrophy due to pressure on the nerves by closure of the foramina. The liver and spleen are enlarged and an element of hypersplenism may occur. Death is usually due to infection, bleeding or anaemia. Recently, bone marrow transplantation has successfully reversed haematologic and bone changes, possibly by supplying functional osteoclasts.

RECOMMENDED READING

Bithell T.C. & Wintrobe M.M. (1967) Drug-induced apalstic anemia. *Seminars in Hematology* **4**, 194.

Bottiger L.E. & Westerholm B. (1972) Aplastic anaemia III. Aplastic anaemia and infectious hepatitis. *Acta medica Scandinavia* **192**, 323.

Camitta B.M., Nathan D.G., Forman E.N., Parkman R., Rappoport S. & Orellana T. (1974) Posthepatitic severe aplastic anemia. An indication for early bone marrow transplantation. *Blood* **43**, 473.

Coccia P.F., Krivit W., Cervenka J. *et al.* (1980) Successful bone marrow transplantation for infantile malignant osteopetrosis. *New England Journal of Medicine* **302**, 701.

Diamond L.K., Allen D.M. & Magill F.B. (1961) Congenital (erythroid) hypoplastic anemia. *American Journal of Diseases of Childhood* **102**, 403.

Estren S. & Dameshek W. (1947) Familial hypoplastic anaemia of childhood. Report of eight cases in two families with beneficial effect of splenectomy in one case. *American Journal of Diseases of Childhood* **73**, 671.

Fanconi G. (1967) Familial constitutional panmyelocytopathy, Fanconi's anemia. *Seminars in Hematology* **4**, 233.

Fitchem J.H. & Cline M.J. (1978) Recent developments in understanding the pathogenesis of aplastic anemia. *American Journal of Hematology* **5**, 365.

Gordon-Smith E.C. (1972) Bone-marrow failure: diagnosis and treatment. *British Journal of Haematology* **13**, Suppl., 167.

Krantz S.B. (1974) Pure red cell aplasia. *New England Journal of Medicine* **291**, 345.

Li F.P., Alter B.P. & Nathan D.G. (1972) The mortality of acquired aplastic anemia in children. *Blood* **40**, 153.

O'Gorman Hughes D.W. (1969) Aplastic anaemia in childhood: a reappraisal. I. Classification and assessment. *Medical Journal of Australia* **I**, 1059.

Peschle C., Marmont A.M., Marone G., Genovese A., Sasso G.F. & Condorelli M. (1975) Pure red cell aplasia: studies on an IgG serum inhibitor neutralising erythropoietin. *British Journal of Haematology* **30**, 522.

Stohlman F., Jr (1972) Aplastic anemia (Editorial). *Blood* **40**, 282.

Storb R. & Thomas E.D. (1975) Bone marrow transplantation for aplastic anaemia. *British Journal of Haematology* **31**, suppl., 83.

Symposium (1978) *Clinical Hematology* 7, 431.

Thomas E.D. *et al.* (1972) Aplastic anaemia treated by marrow transplantation. *Lancet* **I**, 184.

Zaentz S.D., Krantz S.B. & Brown E.B. (1976) Studies on pure red cell aplasia. VIII. Maintenance therapy with immunosuppressive drugs. *British Journal of Haematology* **32**, 47.

Worlledge S.M. (1973) Immune drug-induced hemolytic anemias. *Seminars in Hematology* **10**, 327.

Chapter 12
Haemolytic Anaemias

Red cells normally survive approximately 120 days (80 days in the neonate). Haemolytic anaemia occurs when there is shortened survival of red cells due to their premature destruction. Destruction occurring in excess of production results in anaemia.

The causes of haemolytic anaemia are probably best classified according to the mechanism of premature red cell destruction. These are divided into disorders which are intrinsic to the red cells and those due to extrinsic factors:

Intrinsic defects

1 Red cell membrane disorders.
(a) Hereditary spherocytosis.
(b) Hereditary elliptocytosis.
(c) Hereditary stomatocytosis.
2 Enzyme disorders.
(a) Pentose phosphate pathway abnormalities (G6PD, glutathione synthetase, etc.).
(b) Glyocolytic enzyme deficiencies (pyruvate kinase, glucose phosphate isomerase, etc.).
3 Haemoglobin abnormalities.
(a) Thalassaemias.
(b) Haemoglobinopathies (Hb, S, E, C, etc.).
(c) Unstable haemoglobins.

Extrinsic causes

1 Immune.
(a) Isoantibodies, causing haemolytic disease of the newborn.
(b) Autoimmune haemolytic anaemia (IgG or 1gM antibodies).
(c) Drug related (penicillin, methyl dopa).
2 Toxins (bacterial, snake venoms, burns).
3 Parasitic infections (malaria, etc.).
4 Microangiopatic haemolytic anaemia.
(a) DIC.
(b) Haemolytic uraemic syndrome.
(c) Miscellaneous (cardiac, carcinoma).

Red cell and haemoglobin catabolism

The exact mechanism of normal red cell destruction is not precisely known. It is probable that as the cells grow older their ability to use glucose to generate ATP decreases due to a gradual failure of the glycolytic enzyme system. This leads to the cells losing their ability to maintain cation balance, leading to accumulation of water. The cells become spherical, lose their elasticity and are trapped in the spleen, liver and bone marrow.

Other mechanisms are almost certainly involved, e.g. mechanical destruction, destruction by reticuloendothelial tissue or loss by bleeding. In all probability, the latter factors play a minor part in normal red cell destruction.

Haemoglobin released by the red cell destruction is broken down in the phagocytes of the reticuloendothelial system. The globin is split off from haem and its components returned to the general metabolic pool. The haem molecule is broken down to form biliverdin and carbon monoxide. The biliverdin is reduced to bilirubin, which is coupled to glucuronic acid by the liver and excreted in the bile. The iron released from the haem molecule enters the body pool for reutilization.

Clinical features of haemolytic anaemia

Patients with haemolytic anaemia may present at any age. Haemolysis is suspected if the patient exhibits anaemia together with evidence of increased red cell destruction, e.g. jaundice, haemoglobinuria.

Acute haemolytic anaemia The symptoms usually have a rapid onset. The symptoms are fever, headache, abdominal and back pain, plus vomiting. The urine may be dark due to free haemoglobin, but, occasionally, oliguria or anuria may be present. The spleen is usually palpable 2 or 3 cm below the costal margin, but the liver and lymph nodes are of normal size.

Chronic haemolytic anaemia usually presents as anaemia with a mild persisting jaundice. The urine contains urobilinogen and haemosiderin can be found when the urine is stained for iron.

Diagnostic approach to suspected haemolytic anaemia

The age at presentation gives a major clue to the likely diagnosis and influences the laboratory investigations.

NEWBORN PERIOD

Important points in the history Obstetric history of mother and child. Family history — possible haemolytic anaemia in other family members. Age of onset of symptoms in relation to birth. Sex of child. Drug history of mother and child.

CHILDREN AFTER NEWBORN PERIOD

Important points in the history Age of onset, sex of child, racial origin. History of haemolysis in the newborn period. Family history of anaemia. Description of symptoms (type of onset, possible acute exacerbations). Drug, food or dietary history. History of travel.

PHYSICAL EXAMINATION

Search for Pallor of the skin. Jaundice, best seen in the sclera. Physical development, skeletal development, splenomegaly, hepatomegaly, adenopathy, purpura or pigmentation.

Laboratory investigations

PRELIMARY INVESTIGATIONS

Tests to confirm the presence of haemolysis which may give a clue to the aetiology: Haemoglobin, leucocyte count, platelet count, reticulocyte count, red cell parameters. Examination of blood film, looking for spherocytosis, agglutination, fragmentation, parasites, inclusion bodies. Plasma haptoglobin, Schumm's test, plasma haemoglobin, bilirubin (conjugated and unconjugated). Direct and indirect antiglobin test. Specificity of any antibody found. Urine examination (urobilinogen, haemoglobin, haemosiderin).

DIRECTED SPECIAL INVESTIGATIONS

Some of these tests will be required to determine the exact aetiology of the haemolysis. The diagnostic tests and ancillary tests for the various haemolytic disorders are listed below:

Hereditary spherocytosis Osmotic fragility and autohaemolysis studies. Sodium influx studies. Family studies.

Hereditary elliptocytosis Blood film. Autohaemolysis is occasionally abnormal. Rh grouping.

Hereditary stomatocytosis Blood film, wet preparation. Sodium influx studies. Calcium influx studies. Intracellular sodium, potassium, calcium and water levels.

Enzyme disorders G6PD screen. Enzyme assays, kinetic studies of abnormal enzyme activity.

Haemoglobinopathies Haemoglobin electrophoresis. Alkali denaturation. Sickle cell preparation. Hb-H preparation. Heinz body preparation. Heat stability test, isopropanol precipitation. Membrane lipid peroxidation. Peptide mapping of abnormal haemoglobins.

Immune haemolysis Direct and indirect antiglobulin test, antibody specificity. Cold agglutinins. Donath-Landsteiner test. Drug related indirect antiglobulin tests. LE test, Ham's test, mycoplasma antibody tests, VDRL. Paul-Bunnell test. Plasma haemoglobin, methaemalbumin.

Parastic infections Thin and thick film for malaria, malarial antibodies. Wet film for filaria. Bone marrow for Kala-Azar.

Microangiopathic haemolytic anaemias Blood coagulation studies. Urine haemosiderin.

Miscellaneous associated studies which may be helpful Serum complement levels. Vitamin E assay. Red cell survival studies. Skeletal X-rays.

MEMBRANE DISORDERS

HEREDITARY SPHEROCYTOSIS

Inheritance

Autosomal dominant disorder with an incidence of about 1 in 5000. A proportion of patients (10—15%) appear to be sporadic.

Pathogenesis

The nature of the membrane defect is unknown, but there is an increased influx of sodium across the cell membrane. The lipid content of the red cell membrane is decreased in spite of increased membrane lipid turnover. The glycolytic activity of the red cell is increased and provides the increased amounts of ATP required to maintain increased cation pump activity.

Following exit from the marrow, the red cells assume a spherical shape. In this state, they are less deformable than normal biconcave red cells and become trapped in the sinuses of the spleen. Here, they become depleted of glucose stores, their ATP level drops and the eflux of Na^+ cannot be maintained. Lysis occurs as a result of the influx of water into the cell.

Clinical features

The severity of symptoms is variable, ranging from severe haemolysis in the newborn period with hyperbilirubinaemia requiring exchange transfusion to symptoms of a mild chronic anaemia which may be associated with bouts of abdominal pain, or even asymptomatic spherocytosis, often found by accident when the blood film is examined for other reasons or as part of a family study.

Haemolytic crises may occur, especially with infections, causing an increase in the anaemia and jaundice. Rarely aplastic crises may occur, as characterized by severe pallor, marked symptoms of anaemia and lessening of jaundice. Investigations show an absence of reticulocytes with bone marrow erythroblastopenia.

Physical findings

Splenomegaly is a characteristic finding. Liver and lymph nodes are not usually enlarged. Jaundice and pallor may be clinically apparent.

Laboratory tests

The haemoglobin level is often decreased, but the MCHC is high (>35 g/dl). Spherocytes are seen on the blood film, often in large numbers. Occasionally, the spherocytes may be difficult to find. The osmotic fragility is increased in hypotonic saline solutions, an effect which is accentuated by 24 hours of incubation at 37°C. The autohaemolysis is increased after incubation for 48 hours at 37°C, but is corrected by the addition of glucose. The red cell sodium influx is increased to about 50% above normal values.

Differential diagnosis of spherocytosis seen on blood film examination

Newborns usually have a small number of spherocytes present, which disappear within the first few months after birth. Diagnosis in this period may be difficult, but examination of the parents' blood film may be of help.

Haemolysis due to autoimmune haemolytic anaemia, isoimmune haemolysis, G6PD deficiency and other enzyme abnormalities, infantile pyknocytosis and burns, can be associated with spherocytosis on blood film examination. Appropriate histories and laboratory tests will distinguish hereditary spherocytosis from these conditions.

Treatment

Splenectomy decreases the rate of haemolysis and returns red cell survival to almost normal levels. However, splenectomy may be followed by severe infections, particulary in young children. The need for splenectomy can be assessed by the following indications:

1 Positive family history of splenectomy.
2 Recurrent haemolytic crises.
3 Recurrent aplastic crises.
4 History and/or evidence of pigment gallstones.

If **2**, **3** or **4** are present, splenectomy should be performed as soon as it is feasible. If there is only a positive family history splenectomy, then the operation should be postponed until the child has had 1–2 years of primary schooling. In sporadic cases, or when there is a negative family history of splenectomy, it may be reasonable to avoid splenectomy altogether, provided that haemolysis is well compensated and the patient is asymptomatic. The presence of pigment stones, demonstrated by ultrasound examination of the gallbladder, is an indication for splenectomy in these patients. This investigation should be performed in all patients considered for splenectomy.

Folic acid (5 mg/week) should be given to children with hereditary spherocytosis, as there is an increased rate of erythropoiesis which may deplete folic acid stores. Haemolytic and aplastic crises may require blood transfusion, but transfusion is otherwise rarely required.

HEREDITARY ELLIPTOCYTOSIS

Hereditary elliptocytosis is a common disorder, with an incidence of about 1 in 2500. The majority of patients with elliptocytosis do not have haemolysis. About 12% of patients have mild compensated haemolysis. Uncompensated haemolysis is very uncommon. An increased number (25–90%) of oval elliptical or elongated red cells are noted on the blood film.

The disorder is inherited as an autosomal dominant. Homozygous inheritance in patients has been described, with severe haemolytic anaemia dating from birth.

The disorder must be distinguished from other causes of elliptocytosis. Megaloblastic anaemia has oval cells which are macrocytic. Elliptocytes are also seen in iron deficiency, thalassaemia and associated with marrow replacement.

No active treatment is required.

HEREDITARY STOMATOCYTOSIS

This is a group of conditions with altered cation flux across the cell membrane. Examination of the blood film shows that up to 50% of the red cells have a slit (stoma) instead of the usual round central pallor. In wet preparations, the fixed red cells are crucible shaped instead of biconcave discs. Inheritance appears to be autosomal dominant in some cases, while in other patients the mode of inheritance is not certain.

Clinically, patients vary in the severity of haemolysis. The flux of sodium and potassium irons across the cell membrane is increased and there are variations of the intracellular cation concentrations.

Transfusions are occasionally required when severe haemolysis exists. Splenectomy is variably successful in relieving symptoms of haemolysis.

ACANTHOCYTOSIS

This disorder is characterized by the presence of spherical red cells with projecting spikes — 'spur cells'. It may be primary or secondary in aetiology.

PRIMARY

Haemolytic anaemia is associated with absence of β-lipoproteins, usually inherited as an autosomal recessive disorder. The predominant features of the disorder are not haematological. Patients develop ataxia due to degeneration of cerebellar, posterior column and pyramidal tracts. Steatorrhoea, retinitis pigmentosa and growth retardation are part of the disease complex. The anaemia is mild.

SECONDARY

Ususally due to liver disease with low levels of β-lipoprotein.

The haematological effects of secondary acanthocytosis are usually more severe, with obvious haemolysis and splenomegaly. Factors such as nutrition may play a part in the production of haemolysis.

Differential diagnosis

Spur cells can also be seen in vitamin E deficiency, some enzyme disorders (e.g. PK and GPI deficiencies) and associated with the McLeod red cell phenotype (cells lacking the Kell antigen).

VITAMIN E DEFICIENCY (INFANTILE PYKNOCYTOSIS)

Haemolytic anaemia due to low levels of vitamin E may occur in newborn infants. The babies are usually premature and of low birth weight (usually < 1.5 kg).

Vitamin E is an anti-oxidant and, in the neonate, is thought to prevent oxidation of the red cell membrane at a time when there is a physiological deficiency of the enzyme glutathione peroxidase. Oxidation of lipid double bonds on cell membranes is accelerated by the presence of ferrous and cuprous ions, and this is inhibited by vitamin E, which acts as a scavenger for free radicals.

Additional factors appear to be operative in the production of infantile pyknocytosis. These are: increased amounts of polyunsaturated fats in artificial milk formulas increase the tendency of the red cell membrane lipids to oxidation; malabsorption of vitamin E; low body stores of vitamin E; the administration of iron as prophylaxis against iron deficiency anaemia due to prematurity.

Clinical features

The babies usually are premature and/or of low birth weight. The haemoglobin level is low, with values as low as 5 g/dl being occasionally found. There is reticulocytosis up to 10%, the bilirubin is slightly to moderately elevated. The blood film shows contracted spiky red cells (pyknocytes) as well as normal red cells. The peroxide lysis test is positive and the assay of serum vitamin E levels shows values less than 5 μg/ml.

Treatment

In many centres, vitamin E is given prophylactically to all infants with a birth weight of less than 2.5 kg. The dose is 20–40 mg/day. Prophylactic iron is not commenced until the infants are 2 months old. Treatment for established pyknocytosis is with α-tocopherol 40 mg/day. The normal daily requirement is 0.5 mg for breast-fed babies and 1.5 mg for babies on artificial feeds. Response to therapy is good, no evidence of the disorder being seen beyond 6–12 months of age. Disappearance of the pyknocytes from the blood film may be delayed well beyond the cessation of the haemolysis.

ENZYME DISORDERS

Energy for the maintenance of red cell integrity is obtained by metabolism of glucose. Two inter-related systems are involved in the catabolism of the glucose to lactate, the Embden-Meyerhof pathway (EMP) and the aerobic hexose monophosphate pathway (HMP).

About 90% of glucose passes through the Embden-Meyerhof pathway. Each mole of glucose is catabolized to two moles of lactate, with a net gain of two moles of ATP. Of the 13 enzymes involved in this pathway, seven have well documented abnormalities associated with chronic nonspherocytic haemolytic anaemia. These are:

1 Hexokinase (HK).
2 Glucose phosphate isomerase (GPI).
3 Phosphofructokinase (PFK).
4 Triose phosphate isomerase (TPI).
5 Phosphoglycerate kinase (PGK).
6 2,3-diphosphoglycerate mutase (2,3-DPGM).
7 Pyruvate kinase (PK).

With three other enzymes, glyceraldehyde phosphate dehydrogenase (GAPD), 2,3-diphosphoglycerate phosphatase (2,3-DPGP) and enolase, there is not a clear link between metabolic effects of enzyme abnormalities described and haemolysis in the patients. All of these enzyme abnormalities are rare.

The hexose monophosphate pathway uses about 10% of the glucose metabolized by red cells. The first step involves the enzyme, glucose-

6-phosphate-dehydrogenase (G6PD). A large number of abnormalities of this enzyme have been described, and in excess of 100 million people are affected throughout the world.

GLUCOSE-6-PHOSPHATE-DEHYDROGENASE DEFICIENCY

Deficiency occurs in four broad ethnic groups: (1) Africans, (2) Mediterranean and Middle Eastern, (3) South-East Asian and (4) a miscellaneous group. The first three groups account for the vast majority of people with the enzyme abnormality, suffering sporadic episodes of haemolysis. The haemolytic crises are associated with drug ingestion (see list below), infections (bacterial and viral infections), hepatitis and ketoacidosis. In addition, the Mediterranean group experiences haemolysis following the eating of broad beans (vicia faba).

The miscellaneous group represents a small group of patients with variant G6PD enzymes (in excess of 100 variants have been described). Some of these patients have a chronic haemolytic anaemia, while others have no clinical evidence of haemolysis. The G6PD variant enzymes show a variety of kinetic and physiochemical properties.

The enzyme exists as either a two or four subunit molecule with a total MW of 200 000. Two enzymes with normal activity and stability exist, the B+ and the A+. The A+ enzyme results from the substitution of a single amino acid in the molecule (aspartic acid in A+ for asparagine in B+). The B+ enzyme is present in all Caucasians and in 70% of Africans. About 30% of the Africans have the A+ enzyme, which has faster electrophoretic mobility.

G6PD acts to convert glucose-6-phosphate to 6-phosphogluconate, the first step in the hexose monophate shunt (Fig. 12.1). During this reaction, NADP is reduced to NADPH, which subsequently is involved in a variety of reactions necessary to maintain the normal reduced state of the cytoplasmic and membrane constituents of the red cell. The decreased ability of the G6PD deficient cell to resist oxidation is the cause of the haemolysis.

Ten to 15% of African negroes suffer haemolytic episodes due to G6PD abnormality, the variant G6PD being termed A–. This enzyme has the same electrophoretic mobility as the A+ enzyme, but is unstable *in vivo* and its total enzyme activity is reduced to 10–20% of the normal levels. The activity decreases as the red cell ages, so that younger red cells have higher activity than older cells.

G6PD related haemolytic anaemia occurring in people from the Mediterranean area, is usually due to the enzyme varient, G6PD Mediterranean. This isoenzyme has very low activity (0–7%) and is very unstable. In the Asian area, a variety of isoenzymes occur, the commonest being G6PD Canton.

Fig. 12.1 Action of G6PD.

$$\text{G6P} + \text{NADP} \xrightarrow{\text{G6PD}} \text{6PG} + \text{NADPH}$$

The gene for G6PD is carried on the X chromosome. Defective genes affect hemizygous males and homozygous females. Heterozygous females usually have enzyme activity which is lower than normal, and two populations of cells can be demonstrated by staining procedures — one with normal activity, the other showing decreased activity.

Clinical features

Four clinical syndromes occur associated with G6PD deficiency: (1) neonatal haemolysis, (2) favism, (3) drug-induced haemolysis and (4) chronic haemolytic anaemia.

NEONATAL HAEMOLYSIS

Severe jaundice occurring in the newborn with G6PD deficiency has been widely reported. The jaundice usually begins between the second and the fifth day after birth. There is no isoimmune cause for the haemolysis and, frequently, no precipitating cause can be found. There is a marked anaemia with a high reticulocyte count. The haemolysis usually lasts 1–2 weeks. Exchange transfusion is often required to prevent kernicterus.

FAVISM

Acute haemolysis occurs following eating of broad beans or inhaling its pollen. It is more likely to occur after eating fresh or raw beans than old or well cooked beans. Inhalation of pollen may produce haemolysis within minutes. Patients with favism mostly have G6PD Mediterranean, but it has also been reported in the Chinese and in patients with G6PD Zähringen. Favism does not occur in negroes.

Haemolysis begins within hours of ingestion of the beans. There is a precipitous fall in haemoglobin, with jaundice and haemoglobinuria. Emergency transfusion is often necessary. Unidentified additional factors appear to be involved in the inheritance of sensitivity to broad beans.

DRUG-INDUCED HAEMOLYSIS

Acute haemolysis follows ingestion of a large group of drugs which can cause oxidation of red cell components. In addition, acute haemolysis may follow acute bacterial and viral infections and ketoacidosis. The drugs which invariably cause haemolysis are listed in the left hand column of Table 12.1. Drugs which have been given in association with fevers, but are not clearly causative, are listed in the right-hand column.

The haemolysis begins within 3 days of drug ingestion. There is usually marked haemolysis with anaemia and haemoglobinuria. The haemoglobin may fall to extremely low levels, requiring transfusion.

CHRONIC HAEMOLYTIC ANAEMIA

Of the nearly 100 variant G6PDs described, about 35 are associated with chronic haemolysis of a mild to severe nature. Increased haemolysis occurs with fever, exposure to oxidant drugs and, occasionally, broad beans. The isoenzymes vary in physiochemical properties. The interested reader is referred to larger texts for detailed information. This group is relatively rare in comparison to other groups of G6PD deficient patients.

Table 12.1 Drugs associated with haemolysis in G6PD deficiency.

Causative drugs	May cause haemolysis if associated with fever
Antimalarials	
Primaquine	Chloroquine
Pamaquine	Quinine*
Quinocide	Quinacrine
Pantaquine	
Analgesics	
Acetanilide	Acetylsalicylic acid
Antipyrine*	Acetophenetidin
Aminopyrine*	*p*-Aminosalicylic acid
Sulphonamides	Sulphadiazine
Salicylazosulphapyridine	
Sulphapyridine	Sulphamerazine
Sulphamethoxypyridazine	Sulphoxone
N-Acetylsulphanilamide	Sulphathiazole
Thiazolesulphone	
Miscellaneous	
Phenylhydrazine	Aniline
Acetylphenylhydrazine	Antazolene
Napthalene	Ascorbic acid
Sulphones	Chloramphenicol*
Nalidixic acid	Dimercaprol
Neoarsphenamine	Diphenhydramine
Toluidine blue	Methylene blue
Nitrobenzene	*p*-Aminophenol
Trinitrotoluene	*p*-Aminobenzoic acid
Fava beans	Procaine amide
	Probenecid
	Pyrimethamine
	Vitamin K (water-soluble analogues)

**Described in Caucasians only.*

Laboratory diagnosis

In the non-haemolytic state, the haemoglobin and blood film are normal. During haemolysis, the haemoglobin often falls to very low levels (5 g/dl). The red cells are often spherocytic, many cells showing an area on one side which does not contain haemoglobin (blister cell). Heinz bodies are seen in the 1–2 days prior to the commencement of the haemolysis, but are uncommon once haemolysis has begun.

Screening tests rely on the ability of the red cells to produce NADPH. The NADPH is then used to decolourize dyes (brilliant cresyl blue), reduce methaemoglobin or is detected by its ability to fluoresce.

Assay of G6PD activity is performed by observing the rate of production of NADPH from NADP. Mediterranean and oriental patients have very low levels of activity (undetectable to 7%), while negro hemizygote males have 3–15% of normal activity. Occasionally, patients in haemolytic crisis may have G6PD activity at normal or near normal levels due to the presence of a large proportion of young cells which have a high enzyme content. If an older population of red cells cannot be obtained for assay by differential centrifugation, measurement of enzyme activity may have to be delayed until the patient's red cells have aged.

Treatment

Avoidance of precipitating situations (drugs, fevers, eating broad beans, etc.) should be stressed with susceptible patients. Exchange transfusions of affected neonates with haemolysis may be required to prevent kernicterus. Transfusion of patients with haemolytic crisis is usually necessary.

NON-SPHEROCYTIC HAEMOLYTIC ANAEMIAS

Abnormalities of a number of the enzymes of the Embden-Meyerhof pathway and the hexose phosphate pathway result in a group of patients with continuous haemolytic anaemia. Numerically, they are uncommon, with pyruvate kinase (PK) deficiency being the most common. The remainder of enzyme abnormalities are rare, but are important because of their metabolic significance and the severity of the conditions produced in the patients with the disorders. A list of the enzyme deficiencies associated with haemolytic anaemias is given in Table 12.2.

PYRUVATE KINASE

Pyruvate kinase deficiency is inherited as an autosomal recessive and has been reported from all over the world. Homozygotes have from 10–20% of normal enzyme activity, with intermediate activity of heterozygotes. Approximately 1% of the population are heterozygous.

Clinical features

The severity of the symptoms shows great variation, from a severe haemolytic anaemia presenting in the neonatal period to a mild compensated haemolysis diagnosed during adult life. Jaundice, hepatomegaly and a high incidence of gallstones occur in patients with marked haemolysis, accompanied by slight to moderate splenomegaly. Skeletal changes are uncommon and, when present, consist of frontal bossing.

The degree of anaemia is variable, haemoglobin values varying from 4–12 g/dl. The oxygen affinity of the patient's blood is reduced because of raised levels of 2,3-DPG, so that oxygen is released from the haemoglobin molecule more readily than normal. The result is a lessening of the effect of the anaemia found in these patients. Increased haemolysis occurs with infections and rarely an aplastic crisis may occur.

Laboratory diagnosis

Prior to splenectomy, the red cells do not shown any characteristic morphology. A reticulocytosis of from 5 to 10% may increase to over 50% after splenectomy. Splenectomy is followed by the appearance of a large number of 'spiky' spherocytes in the blood film.

Osmotic fragility is normal with unincubated blood and is usually normal after 24 hours of incubation, although it may occasionally be increased. The result of autohaemolysis is variable; typically, there is increased haemolysis which is not corrected by added glucose. The addition of high concentrations of ATP corrects the haemolysis in this test by an unknown mechanism.

Table 12.2 Enzyme deficiencies associated with haemolytic anaemia.

Embden-Myerhof pathway
Hexokinase
Glucose phosphate isomerase
Phosphofructokinase
Aldolase
Triose phosphate isomerase
2, 3-Diphosphoglycerate mutase
Phosphoglycerate kinase
Pyruvate kinase
Hexose monophosphate shunt
Glucose-6-phosphate dehydrogenase
γ-glutamyl-cysteine synthetase
Glutathione synthetase
Non-glycolytic enzyme deficiencies
Adenylate kinase
Pyrimidine 5-nucleotidase

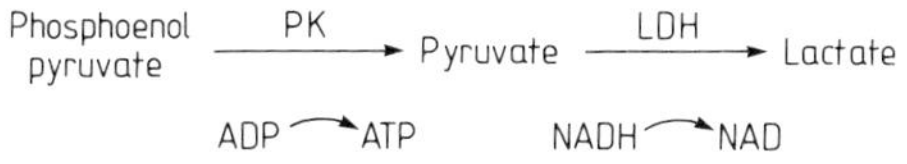

Fig. 12.2 Biochemical basis of PK enzyme assay.

A fluorescent screening test is available. Assay of red cell enzyme activity is performed by coupling the reaction to the formation of lactate and monitoring the rate of oxidation of NADH to NAD (see Fig. 12.2).

A large number of isoenzymes have been found, with differing activity for substrates, rate of reaction, etc. It may be necessary to assess heat stability and perform kinetic studies before the correct level of enzyme activity can be estimated. Leucocytes have high activity, so that removal of leucocytes prior to assay is essential. The biochemical effects of the abnormality are complicated and the reader is referred to larger texts, but haemolysis appears to be related to reduced amounts of ATP produced by the cells.

Treatment

Blood transfusions are given as required for symptomatic relief of haemolytic or aplastic crises. Splenectomy often produces an improvement in patients who have marked haemolysis by reducing the rate of haemolysis and decreasing the need for transfusion. Cholecystectomy for cholelithiasis is often necessary in the second or later decades.

EXTRINSIC CAUSES OF HAEMOLYTIC ANAEMIA

IMMUNE HAEMOLYTIC ANAEMIA

The destruction of red cells following the attachment of antibodies of their surfaces gives rise to immune haemolytic anaemia. The antibodies may pass from the mother via the placenta to the child to produce haemolytic disease of the newborn — isoimmune haemolytic anaemia. Alternately, the antibodies may be produced by the patient, either spontaneously or following a variety of stimuli, and cause premature destruction of red blood cells — autoimmune haemolytic anaemia (AIHA).

The antibodies produced vary in their characteristics and their mode of action. Antibodies which react best at 37°C are termed 'warm' antibodies and, in general, are IgG molecules. One type of IgG antibody reacts best at 4°C, causing the attachment of complement to the red cell, a condition called paroxysmal cold haemoglobinuria. A second group of antibodies reacts best at temperatures below 20°C, and are called 'cold' antibodies, these being IgM molecules. Rarely, IgA antibodies are produced by the patient and behave as 'warm' antibodies.

AUTOIMMUNE HAEMOLYTIC ANAEMIA (AIHA)

Autoimmune haemolytic anaemia occurs following the production by the patient of antibodies which react with their own red cells. They are either 'warm' (IgG) or 'cold' (IgM) antibodies. Attachment of the antibodies to the surface of the red cells leads to their premature destruction by the reticuloendothelial tissue or to their lysis in the blood stream.

A state of compensated haemolysis may occur if an increase in marrow red cell output can match the rate of their destruction. Anaemia results if destruction exceeds the ability of the marrow to produce new red cells.

Classification

Classification may be according to the type of antibody produced — warm (IgG), cold (IgM), paroxysmal cold haemoglobinuria (IgG) or according to the aetiology. One such classification is shown in Table 12.3.

Antibodies and mechanisms of haemolysis

The most common antibodies are of the IgG class. They have a MW of 160 000, are heat stable and react best at 37°C (warm antibodies).

Table 12.3 Classification of AIHA.

Cause	Type of antibody	Temperature range of antibody test
Idiopathic	IgG	Warm
Drug-induced		
Methyldopa	IgG	Warm
Penicillin	IgG	Drug dependent agglutination or lysis in presence of complement
Stibophen	IgG	Drug dependent agglutination or lysis in presence of complement
Infections		
Cytomegalovirus	IgG	Warm
Hepatitis	IgG	Warm
Infectious mononucleosis	IgM	Cold
Mycoplasma	IgM	Cold
Paroxysmal cold haemoglobinuria	IgG	Donath-Landsteiner test
Associated diseases		
'Autoimmune'	IgG	Warm
Immunodeficiency	IgG	Warm
Lymphoma	IgM	Cold

Approximately 35% of patients have IgG alone attached to the red cells, while 40% have both IgG and complement attached. In a small proportion of patients (10%), complement is detected without IgG antibody. The IgG often shows specificity for one of the Rh antigens, commonly the *e* antigen. A proportion of the antibodies is directed against the Rh 'core' antigen. It is rare for this type of antibody to be directed against other blood group antigens.

In children, an occasional IgG antibody is detected with specificity for the red cell P antigen. This antibody reacts best at 4°C and binds complement. Upon warming, the antibody detaches from the red cells, while the complement remains, causing marked haemolysis. This haemolytic disorder is called paroxysmal cold haemoglobinuria. The presence of this antibody is detected by the Donath-Landsteiner test.

Destruction of the sensitized red cells occurs mainly in the spleen. Intravascular haemolysis is uncommon in 'warm' AIHA, although it may be a feature in the acute phase. The macrophages of the spleen recognize the Fc fragment of the IgG molecule coating the red cells and either phagocytose the entire cell or destroy a portion of the cell membrane, leaving a spherocytic red cell which is vulnerable to subsequent destruction on its return to the spleen.

Cells coated with the C3b component of complement are thought to be recognized by the liver macrophages which neutralize the C3b, leaving C3d on the cell surface. These cells are then phagocytosed by the reticulo-endothelial cells.

Intravascular haemolysis may occur following the activation of the complement system to its completion. It is not understood why the most cases of 'warm' AIHA do not progress to complete complement activation.

IgM antibodies are large molecules (MW $\simeq 10^6$) which react below 20°C and are termed 'cold' antibodies. They react best at 4°C and are inactive at 37°C. The size of the molecules enables them to bridge the gap between the cells, so that the antibodies are termed 'complete'. They bind complement to the red cell surface which is activated to the C3b stage, causing the cells to be recognized by liver macrophages which initiate red cell destruction.

DRUG INDUCED HAEMOLYSIS

Drug-induced haemolysis occurs following exposure of the patient to some drugs. It is believed that three mechanisms are responsible:

1 The drug may stimulate the production of an antibody which is directed against the drug. Penicillin is such a drug and, following administration, it is absorbed onto the red cell surface where the antibody becomes attached to the drug, leading to the destruction of the red cell. In this situation, the red cell is the innocent bystander.

2 The drug may form a drug-plasma protein complex which is antigenic. This complex binds with antibody and is non-specifically absorbed onto the red cell surface, where it activates complement and causes lysis of the red cell. Drugs such as phenacetin, insulin, antihistamines and stibophen cause haemolysis by this mechanism.

3 A third group of drugs, such as methyldopa, L-dopa and mefenamic acid, induce the production of antibodies in patients. These antibodies are of the IgG class and are active against the Rh antigen. While 15% of the patients receiving methyldopa develop a positive Coombs' test, only about 1% of these patients have active haemolysis.

Clinical features

Idiopathic and secondary AIHA is less common in children than in adults. It is more common in children under the age of 5 years than over that age, with a peak incidence during the first year of life.

The onset is usually acute, with often a history of preceding viral infection or immunization. Marked pallor and jaundice are noted, often accompanied by fever and haemoglobinuria. Symptoms of acute intravascular haemolysis may be present with abdominal pain. Vomiting, diarrhoea, shock and occasionally renal failure may follow.

The symptoms of acute intravascular haemolysis may follow exposure to cold in paroxysmal cold haemoglobinuria. Symptoms of respiratory infection may accompany mycoplasma infection. Splenomegaly is slight to moderate, and hepatomegaly or lymphadenopathy are uncommon.

Chronic haemolytic anaemia is uncommon under the age of 10 years. There is a gradual onset of pallor, with mild jaundice, but haemoglobinuria is usually not present. The spleen may be moderately enlarged.

Laboratory diagnosis

The haemoglobin, haematocrit, reticulocyte count and examination of the blood film constitute initial investigations. The blood film shows spherocytes, red cell fragmentation and agglutination. The pattern of agglutination is often helpful. Warm (IgG) antibodies produce small to moderate size clumps of cells. Cold (IgM) antibodies produce massive agglutination unless the glass slides and blood are kept warm when making the blood film. Erythrophagocytosis is occasionally seen, especially in paroxysmal cold haemoglobinuria. Platelets are usually normal, but are occasionally decreased (Evans' syndrome).

The presence of antibodies on the red cells is detected by the direct antiglobulin (Coombs') test, using both polyspecific antisera directed against IgG, IgM and complement and monospecific antisera. Circulating antibody in the patient's serum is detected by the use of the indirect antiglobulin test, in which the serum of the patient is incubated with Group O, Rh positive cells before testing with antiglobulin sera. The use of the enzyme treated cells enhances the sensitivity of the test.

The specificity of the antibody is determined, either following elution from the red cells of the patient or using the circulating antibody present in the patient's serum. Should the antibody exhibit specificity for a particular red cell antigen, that antigen can often be avoided when providing blood for transfusion.

Detection of cold agglutinins in the serum of patients with IgM antibodies is carried out by incubating the patient's serum, which has been separated at 37°C, with Group O Rh positive cells at 4°C, 20°C, 32°C and 37°C. Other temperatures may be selected to document the range of the thermal activity of the antibody. The titre of the antibody may often be high, levels in excess of 1 in 1 000 000 being occasionally seen. Cold agglutinins most often act against the *i* antigen, found on fetal red cells, especially following infectious mononucleosis.

DONATH-LANDSTEINER TEST

The antibody causing paroxysmal cold haemoglobinuria is an IgG antibody and binds to red cells at 4°C along with complement and, on warming, lysis results following the activation of complement. This series of events can be produced *in vitro* and are called the Donath-Landsteiner test.

Treatment

In the majority of children there is a spontaneous recovery. Treatment is necessary for symptoms of anaemia which may require transfusion. Steroids are usually required in the acute phase if there is a need to transfuse the patient. Splenectomy may be required for severe and persistent haemolysis.

TRANSFUSION

Transfusion is used when there are symptoms from the anaemia or a progressive rapid fall in haemoglobin. It should be undertaken with caution. The presence of circulating antibodies in the serum may make the finding of 'compatible' blood difficult. The blood group specificity of the antibody is determined and, if activity against a specific red cell antigen is found, blood selected for transfusion should lack that antigen.

For example, most IgG antibodies are active against one or all of the Rh antigens; should a specific antigen, such as the *e* antigen, be the target of the antibody, the Rh group of blood selected for transfusion should not contain the *e* antigen, i.e. the blood should be *EE* phenotype. If no antibody specificity can be demonstrated, the blood issued for transfusion should be no more incompatible with the patient than the patient's own red cells are with his serum, as demonstrated in the autocontrol section of the crossmatch.

Reactions to the transfusions are uncommon and are repeated as required. Should the antibody be more active in the cold, the blood should be warmed to 37°C.

STEROIDS

These are most useful and most often required in patients with warm antibodies. They are seldom useful or required in patients with cold antibodies. The usual dose is 50 mg/m^2 orally daily. The effect of steroids may be monitored with repeated haemoglobin, reticulocyte counts and Coombs' test estimations. A fall in the level of reticulocytes and the conversion of a positive Coombs' test to a negative one are an indication for rapid tapering of the dose of steroids. Usually, tapering of steroids can commence after 2 weeks on full dose and therapy can be discontinued altogether after 4–8 weeks. Persistence of symptoms with a reticulocytosis and positive Coombs' test indicates that autoimmune haemolysis is continuing and that prolonged steroid therapy will be required. The dose of steroids in such patients should be gradually reduced to the minimum compatible with a normal haemoglobin level.

SPLENECTOMY

Splenectomy is seldom required and is reserved for those patients who fail to respond to steroids, or who relapse when the dose that is required to maintain a normal haemoglobin level is such that there are major undesirable steroid side-effects. It may also be required if haemolysis recurs after steroids are discontinued. Some authorities recommend that Cr^{51} survival of autologous red blood cells be estimated prior to splenectomy, to ensure that there is excessive splenic sequestration. This investigation is of greater importance in planning splenectomy in patients with chronic haemolysis than in those with an acute onset and failure to respond to steroids. Splenectomy is successful in about 75% of such patients. The complications of splenectomy and post splenectomy management are described in Chapter 13.

HAEMOLYTIC DISEASE OF THE NEWBORN

This is another example of extrinsic causes of haemolysis which results from transplacental passage of maternal IgG antibody, which attaches to fetal cells causing haemolysis. The subject will be fully dealt with in Chapter 23.

RECOMMENDED READING

BELLINGHAM A.J. (1976) Haemoglobins with altered oxygen affinity. *British Medical Bulletin* **32**, no. 3 234.

BELLINGHAM A.J. & PRANKERD T.A.J. (1975) Hereditary spherocytosis. *Clinics in Hematology* **4**, 139.

BEUTLER E. (1971) Abnormalities of the hexose monophosphate shunt. *Seminars in Hematology* **8**, 311.

BEUTLER E. (1979) Red cell enzyme defects as nondiseases and diseases. *Blood* **54**, 1.

BRAIN M.C. (1969) Hemolytic-uremic syndrome. *Seminars in Hematology* **6**, 162.

BRAIN M.C. (1970) Microangiopathic hemolytic anaemia. *Annual Review of Medicine* **21**, 133.

BUNN H.F., FORGET B.G. & RANNEY H.M. (1977) *Human Hemoglobins.* W.B. Saunders, Philadelphia.

DACIE J.V. (1975) Autoimmune hemolytic anemia. *Archives of Internal Medicine* **135**, 1293.

DE GRUCHY G.C. & GRIMMES A.J. (1972) The nonspherocytic congenital haemolytic anaemias. *British Journal of Haematology* **23**, suppl., 19.

GLADER B.E. & NATHAN D.G. (1975) Haemolysis due to pyruvate kinase deficiency and other glycolytic enzymopathies. *Clinical Hematology* **4**, 123.

JACOBSON L.B., LONGSTRETH G.F. & EDDINGTON T.S. (1973) Clinical and immunologic features of transient cold agglutinin hemolytic anemia. *American Journal of Medicine* **54**, 514.

MARSCH G.W. & LEWIS S.M. (1969) Cardiac hemolytic anemia. *Seminars in Hematology* **6**, 133.

NATHAN D.G. & SHOHET S.B. (1970) Erythrocyte ion transport defects and hemolytic anaemia: 'Hydrocytosis' and 'desciccytosis'. *Seminars in Hematology* **7**, 381.

PIROFSKY B. (1969) *Autoimmunization and the Autoimmune Hemolytic Anemias.* Williams & Wilkins, Baltimore.

SYMPOSIUM (1976) Immune hemolytic anemias. *Seminars in Hematology* (ed. S.N. Swisher) **13**, 247.

TANAKA K.R. & PAGLIA D.E. (1971) Pyruvate kinase deficiency. *Seminars in Hematology* **8**, 367.

TODD D. (1975) Diagnosis of haemolytic states. *Clinics in Hematology* **4**, 63.

VALENTINE W.N. (1971) Disorders associated with Embden-Myerhof pathway and other metabolic pathways. *Seminars in Hematology* **8**, 348.

VALENTINE W.N. (1979) Hemolytic anemia and inborn errors of metabolism. *Blood* **54**, 549.

Chapter 13
Thalassaemias

In recent years, major advances have been made in the understanding of this group of inherited anaemias. In particular, a variety of defects in globin biosynthesis have been characterized at the molecular level and related to the clinical picture.

STRUCTURE OF HAEMOGLOBINS

The haemoglobins are a group of related proteins (globins), to each of which the same prosthetic group haem (an iron-porphyrin complex) is attached. Each globin chain contains a total of about 150 amino acids linked together by peptide bonds to form a polypeptide. There are four important, normally occurring human globin chains, which have been given the letters of the Greek alphabet — α, β, γ and δ. These globins have their own characteristic amino acid sequence, determined by their structural genes situated on chromosome 11 (β, γ and δ) and chromosome 16 (α).

Adult haemoglobin (haemoglobin A)

This is the normal haemoglobin of the adult, comprising about 98% of the total. It consists of 2α and 2β polypeptide chains.

Adult haemoglobin (haemoglobin A) = $\alpha_2\beta_2$

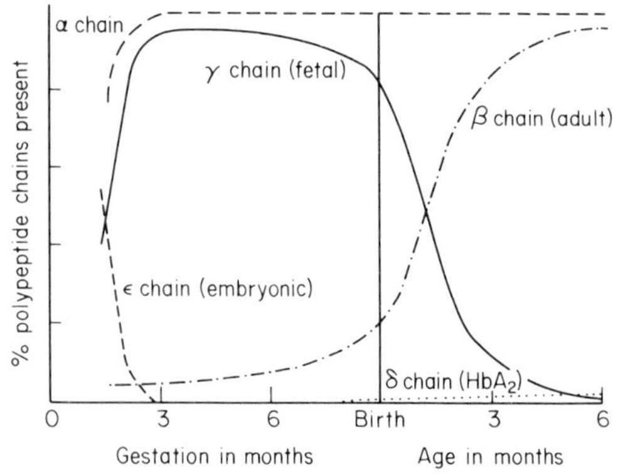

Fig. 13.1 The prenatal and postnatal polypeptide chain presence (from Huehns E.R. 1964).

Small amounts of adult haemoglobin are detectable from about the eighth week post conception. From about the 32nd to 35th week of intrauterine life, this amount normally increases being approximately 10–30% at birth (Fig. 13.1).

Fetal haemoglobin (haemoglobin F)

This is the main type of haemoglobin present during fetal life. It consists of 2α and 2γ chains and has slow electrophoretic mobility. From about 32–36 weeks postconception, the amount gradually decreases so that, at birth, 70–90% of fetal haemoglobin is present. The fetal haemoglobin is virtually all replaced by adult haemoglobin in the first year of life and constitutes less than 2% of the total haemoglobin present in the adult.

Fetal haemoglobin (haemoglobin F) = $\alpha_2\ \gamma_2$

Haemoglobin A_2

This consists of 2α and 2δ chains and has slow electrophoretic mobility. Haemoglobin A_2 begins to appear at the time of birth.

Haemoglobin $A_2 = \alpha_2\ \delta_2$

PATHOGENESIS OF THE THALASSAEMIAS

In the thalassaemias there is decreased or absent production of a specific globin chain. There is a quantitative change in globin production, but no structural change of the affected globin. In β-thalassaemia, there is diminished or absent β globin. In α-thalassaemia, there is diminished or absent α globin. Both β and α thalassaemia result in decreased production of adult haemoglobin.

TYPES OF β-THALASSAEMIA

Heterozygous

This is the most common form of thalassaemia and occurs in two forms, β^+ and β^o. In both, there is usually abnormal red cell morphology with microcytic hypochromic cells and target cells. Associated variations in HbA_2 and HbF are shown in Table 13.1.

Two other disorders, δβ-thalassaemia and hereditary persistence of fetal haemoglobin (HPFH), are related to thalassaemia. In δβ-thalassaemia heterozygotes, there is normal or decreased production of HbA_2 and a higher level of HbF (2–10%) than in β^+- or β^o-thalassaemia. In HPFH, the HbF

Table 13.1 HbA_2 and HbF levels in heterozygous β-thalassaemia.

Type	HbA_2	HbF
β^+-Thalassaemia	Increased	Normal to slightly increased
β^o-Thalassaemia	Increased	Normal to slightly increased
δβ-Thalassaemia	Normal or decreased	Increased (2–10%)
HPFH	Normal or decreased	Increased (10–40%)

production is increased (10–40%) and there is a marked decrease of production of HbA and HbA_2. At a molecular level, δβ-thalassaemia, HPFH and some forms of β^o-thalassaemia are due to gene deletions. The more common β^+-thalassaemia is due to a failure of production of globin mRNA without gene deletion.

In β^+-, β^o- and δβ-thalassaemia, relatively few cells have most of the HbF, and there is a variation in the amount of HbF in different cells, i.e. a 'heterogeneous' distribution whereas, in most cases of HPFH, all cells have relatively equal amounts of HbF, i.e. a 'homogeneous' distribution.

Homozygous

Homozygous β^+-thalassaemia occurs in 1:4 offspring of β^+-heterozygotes. In these patients, there is some detectable β-globin and HbA present. In homozygous β^o-thalassaemia, there are no β-globin or HbA present. In homozygous δβ-thalassaemia, there are no β- or δ-globins and hence no haemoglobin A or A_2; in homozygous HPFH, while there is no HbA or A_2, there are high levels of HbF as, in this condition, there is no 'switch off' of γ chain synthesis after birth.

Although HbF is the major component in both β^+ and β^o homozygous thalassaemia, insufficient amounts are produced to compensate for the decreased production of HbA. As α-globin chains are produced in normal amounts, some will remain unbound to γ or β chains, and these excess α chains precipitate within the cells. There is marked destruction of these cells within the bone marrow and, to a lesser extent, within the spleen, leading to profound anaemia. Anaemia associated with increased erythropoietin levels stimulates ineffective erythropoiesis, resulting in massive erythroid hyperplasia in the bone marrow which can cause bone deformities.

Table 13.2 Types of α-thalassaemia.

Type	Morphology	Ratio of synthesis of α and β-globin chains	Number of α genes
Silent carrier state	Normal	0.8–0.9	3
α-Thalassaemia trait	Abnormal	0.7–0.8	2
HbH disease	Abnormal	0.3–0.6	1
Hydrops fetalis	Abnormal	0	0

TYPES OF α-THALASSAEMIA

There is genetic and biochemical evidence to suggest that there are four α-globin loci per diploid genome and there are four types of α-thalassaemia believed to be related to a loss of function of one to four of these loci (Table 13.2).

Recent work with restriction enzyme gene mapping has demonstrated that the loss of function of the α genes is due, in most cases, to gene deletion.

The silent form is associated with no clinical abnormalities.

α-*Thalassaemia trait* is associated with hypochromia and microcytosis, but no anaemia.

HbH disease arises when excess β-globin chains form unstable tetramers (β_4) which are identifiable by electrophoresis as a rapidly moving haemoglobin band representing 5–30% of the total haemoglobin. This condition is characterized by a chronic haemolytic anaemia with a haemoglobin level of 8–10 g% and associated reticulocytosis. Splenomegaly is usually present. The anaemia may become more severe during pregnancy or infection, or after ingestion of oxidizing drugs which accelerate the precipitation of HbH.

HbBart's hydrops fetalis syndrome is the most severe form of thalassaemia in which no α globin is present and only HbBart's (γ_4) and HbH (β_4) are found. Severe red cell abnormalities are present and the disease is incompatible with postnatal survival. Infants are usually born severely oedematous because of heart failure at 28–36 weeks gestation.

DIAGNOSIS OF MOLECULAR DEFECTS BY GLOBIN CHAIN SYNTHESIS

Globin synthesis can be measured by incubating either peripheral blood (containing reticulocytes) or bone marrow samples with a radioactive amino acid (usually H^3 leucine) and quantitating the amount of radioactivity in α, β and γ chains by column chromatography.

In non-thalassaemic patients, the β/α ratio is close to 1.0. In β^+ and β^o heterozygotes, the β/α ratio is ~0.5. In β^+ homozygotes, the β/α ratio is 0.2–0.04. It is still not known if this variation is due to different levels of β-globin production by different β^+-thalassaemia genes, or to double heterozygosity for β^+ and β^o thalassaemia.

PATHOGENESIS OF ANAEMIA IN THALASSAEMIA

The causes of anaemia in thalassaemia are both primary and secondary.

Primary causes

1 Reduced synthesis of HbA.
2 Ineffective erythropoiesis or intramedullary destruction of erythroid cells.

Secondary causes

1 Folate deficiency.
2 Increasing intravascular volume causing haemodilution.
3 Hypersplenic destruction of red cells.

INCIDENCE

Thalassaemia occurs in people of Mediterranean, South-East Asian, Indian and Middle-Eastern origin. Occasional cases have been described in other ethnic groups, including Anglo-Saxons.

The high incidence in the above racial groups is believed to have resulted from the selective effects of endemic malaria which favoured the propagation of the thalassaemia gene in the heterozygote form. However, it is not known how the heterozygote state for thalassaemia protects against malaria. The variable incidence of malaria may be one of the reasons for the variable incidence of the heterozygotes in different communities, e.g. β-thalassaemia heterozygotes are found in 5% of Italians, 8% of Greeks, 15% of Cypriots and 5% of South-East Asians. Migration has led to a much wider geographical distribution of these disorders. The relatively low incidence of thalassaemia in areas of South-East Asia in which malaria is endemic, has led to the postulate that thalassaemia was brought to Asia by Arab traders.

CLINICAL SYNDROMES

Heterozygous β-thalassaemia (β-thalassaemia minor)

Most people with this condition show no evidence of disease. They may become aware of the diagnosis in one of two ways:
1 By a screening test using red cell indices and blood film, followed by confirmation using haemoglobin electrophoresis or globin chain synthesis (Fig. 13.2);
2 By becoming the parents of a child with homozygous disease. During pregnancy, the extra burden of pregnancy may give rise to additional folate deficiency.

Homozygous β-thalassaemia (β-thalassaemia major)

PRESENTING FEATURES

1 Anaemia usually becomes obvious during the first few months of life, though the severity varies greatly. In some children, it is life-threatening by 3–4 months of age, whereas others are able to maintain the haemoglobin level between 4 and 10 g/100ml for years. Though this is, in part, a haemolytic anaemia, neonatal jaundice is not a feature of this disease.
2 Splenomegaly and hepatomegaly occur and are present earlier in the children with more severe anaemia.

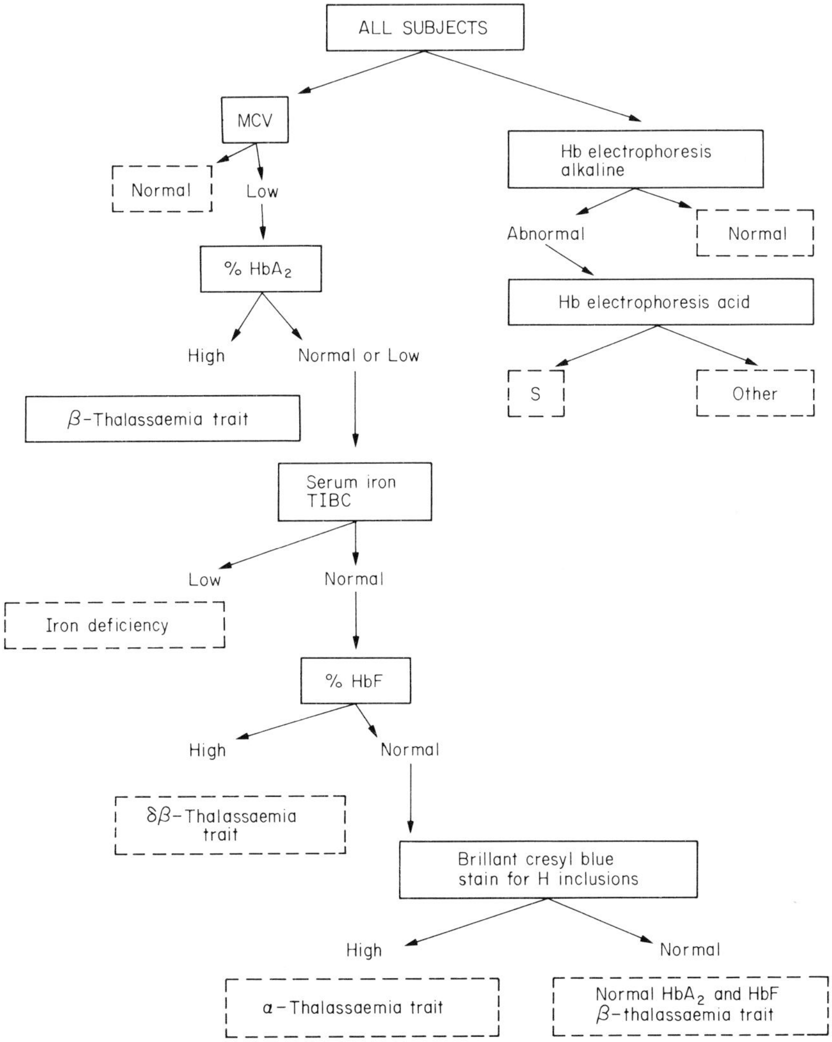

Fig. 13.2 Suggested screening plan (from Alter B. 1979).

3 Bossing of the forehead, prominent cheekbones and protruding upper jaws occur when anaemia has been present for more than a year. These changes are due to expansion of the marrow in the skull and facial bones. Skull X-ray demonstrates the typical 'hair on end' appearance.

4 Rarefaction of long bones is also seen and may be associated with pathological fractures.

DIAGNOSIS

Homozygous β-thalassaemia may be suggested by the severity of the changes in red cell morphology. However, a definite diagnosis may only be made by means of haemoglobin electrophoresis. Globin chain synthesis will differentiate between β^{+}- or β^{o}-thalassaemia. Examination of both parents will determine if the condition is truly homozygous or doubly heterozygous (e.g. $\beta^{+}/\delta\beta$).

COURSE OF THE DISEASE

Modern treatment has altered the course of the disease. However, in the past when minimal transfusions were given, the children developed considerable morbidity from their disease. Below the age of 10 years, the major signs of disease were:

1 Anaemia.

2 Splenomegaly leading to hypersplenism.

3 Frequent intercurrent infections.

4 Gallstones — particularly in children who were able to maintain their haemoglobins, without transfusions, at 6–8 g% for long periods of time.

Above 10 years of age, the main features were:

1 Shortness of stature and delayed puberty.

2 Hepatomegaly with haemosiderosis and disordered liver function.

3 Cardiomegaly related to chronic anaemia and congestive cardiac failure.

4 Cardiac arrhythmias.

5 Endocrine disturbances, particularly diabetes mellitus and hypoparathyroidism.

6 Pericarditis.

CAUSES OF DEATH

Despite changes in management and improved survival, the causes of death remain the same. In young children, the most common cause of death is infection, usually fulminating postsplenectomy infection in children who are not given prophylactic penicillin. In older children, cardiac failure and arrhythmias are the most common cause of death. Diabetes mellitus, hypoparathyroidism and hepatic insufficiency may aggravate these problems.

THALASSAEMIA INTERMEDIA

This term usually refers to a clinical entity which resembles thalassaemia major, but is not as severe. Transfusions are usually not necessary, except at such times as during pregnancy or prior to surgery. Hepatomegaly and splenomegaly are common and splenectomy may become necessary. Cholelithiasis may be present.

With increasing knowledge about the genetic heterogenity of β-thalassaemia, it has become clear that the clinical picture of thalassaemia intermedia can result from a variety of genetic disorders of β chain synthesis. Examples are: homozygous δβ-thalassaemia; doubly heterozygous (β-thalassaemia/silent carrier β-thalassaemia); homozygous β-thalassaemia and α-thalassaemia.

In all of these cases, fetal haemoglobin is always high. Globin chain synthesis studies, particularly on the bone marrow, show a non α/α ratio intermediate between heterozygous and homozygous values. This supports the suggestion that the severity of thalassaemia is attributable to the degree of globin chain synthesis imbalance.

MANAGEMENT

Transfusions

Early transfusion programmes were aimed to raise the haemoglobin to levels which were only sufficient to maintain life. The aim was to minimize iron

Table 13.3 Transfusion programmes.

Programme	Aim
1 Haemoglobin maintained greater than 8 g/100ml	Normal physical activity without symptoms of anaemia Reduced gastrointestinal absorption of iron
2 Haemoglobin raised from 9 g 100ml to 14 g/100ml	Suppression of ineffective erythropoiesis with prevention of splenomegaly, bone changes and gallstones
3 Haemoglobin maintained greater than 12 g/100ml ('super transfusion')	Prevention of cardiomegaly Prevention of expansion of the whole blood volume
4 'Super transfusion' with neocytes or young red cells, i.e. exchange transfusion	Reduction in rate of iron accumulation

loading from transfusions. This type of programme led to long periods of ill-health from anaemia, and the patients suffered from the combined ill-effects of hypoxia and iron overload. Chronic anaemia also caused increased gastrointestinal absorption of iron which, together with iron from the transfusions, resulted in haemosiderosis. Organ failure, particularly of the heart, liver, pancreas and endocrine system, eventually occurred.

Over the last two decades, a number of variations to this programme have been recommended (Table 13.3).

In changing to programmes 1–3, there is an initial increase in the quantity of blood transfused but, once established, the new programme requires an equivalent amount of blood to that in the lower haemoglobin programmes. With a higher average haemoglobin, there is less gastrointestinal absorption of iron and splenomegaly is either delayed or prevented. The effect of the more intensive programmes on the development of organ-failure is not yet known. Programme 4 is yet to be tried in the clinical setting and may prove impractical.

Prior to initiating any transfusion programme, it is essential to obtain a complete genotyping of the patient's red cells. With repeated transfusions, it is possible that both red cell and white cell antibodies may develop. Normally, packed red cells are used for transfusions, but if white cell antibodies develop, buffy coat poor red cells or frozen thawed washed red cells are beneficial.

Blood used for transfusions should be 2–7 days old and hepatitis-antigen negative to avoid infection with hepatitis B and cytomegalovirus. Careful crossmatching is necessary for each transfusion using the patient's blood, which should be collected less than 72 hours before a particular transfusion. Antibodies to the patient's cells or the previous donor's cells may appear at any time.

Complications which may arise during a transfusion, are:

1 Urticarial reactions which require treatment with antihistamines.

2 Febrile reactions which may be due to white cell or plasma protein antibodies. At subsequent transfusion, either buffy coat poor or frozen thawed washed red cells should be used. Antipyretics, such as paracetamol and occasionally steroids, may be necessary.

3 Fluid overload. Most young children can tolerate a flow of 1 unit of blood in 1½ hours, and older children 1 unit in 2 hours. To prevent fluid overload and pulmonary oedema, it is usual to cover the transfusion with a diuretic such as frusemide.

Splenectomy

The main indication for splenectomy is a marked increase in the transfusion requirements, i.e. greater than 50%. The spleen may, to some extent, protect against parenchymal damage from iron overload by extending reticulo-endothelial iron stores, thus preventing deposition of iron in parenchymal cells. However, there comes a point where its destructive effect probably outweighs its value in reducing iron toxicity. After splenectomy, it is wise to withhold transfusion until it has become clear that a patient really cannot do without it, as the operation occasionally unmasks a thalassaemia intermedia.

The risk of fulminating postsplenectomy infection continues indefinitely after splenectomy. Hence, prophylactic penicillin or inoculation with anti pneumococcal and *Haemophilus influenzae* vaccines, is recommended following splenectomy.

Iron chelation therapy

Desferrioxamine binds ferric iron to form ferrioxamine. Oral administration of desferrioxamine results in chelation only of iron already present in the intestine. For chelation of tissue iron, parenteral administration is required. There is evidence to suggest that this binding occurs in both the cells of the reticuloendothelial system and the parenchymal cells of the liver. Once chelated, two-thirds of the ferrioxamine is excreted in the urine and one-third in the stools.

In a few centres in Australia and Britain, routine administration of desferrioxamine by daily intramuscular injection (500–1000 mg) and intravenous infusion (500 mg/unit of blood) has been practised for more than 10 years. Many clinicians, however, have not been prepared to recommend daily injections to their patients because they considered that the relatively small amounts of iron excreted in the urine (6–12 mg in 24 hours) were insufficient. However, reports from centres using regular daily injections of desferrioxamine have claimed the reversal of clinical symptoms and signs of haemosiderosis in the liver and the heart, delay in the accumulation of iron in the liver and prevention of liver fibrosis.

Recently, it has been demonstrated that much higher urinary iron excretions follow intravenous or subcutaneous infusions of desferrioxamine over 10–12 hours. For the first time, negative iron balance seems a possibility and the use of portable battery-operated infusion pumps makes this technically feasible. Most centres favour overnight infusion, as it is less disruptive to the patient's life. Dosage needs to be adjusted for each patient to obtain the maximum iron excretion but, with doses greater than 60 mg/kg body weight, local irritation at the site of the injection may occur. The addition of hydrocortisone (1 mg/ml solution) usually controls this complication.

Vitamin C and desferrioxamine

Although it is recognized that the simultaneous administration of vitamin C with desferrioxamine increases the urinary iron excretion in most patients, increased iron toxicity has been observed in some patients following its introduction. It should therefore be used with caution, if at all.

Folic acid

Folic acid supplements are recommended to prevent the development of relative folic acid deficiency and a megaloblastic crisis which may aggravate the anaemia.

General measures

The medical management of a child with homozygous β-thalassaemia involves good general paediatric and medical care, which includes a close relationship between physician, patient and parents. Anxiety is common amongst children and their parents, so that continuity of care, ease of access to expert medical advice and time for discussion are enormously important. Where more than one child in a family is affected, this imposes an enormous burden on the family. Delayed puberty may cause much psychological distress. Interruptions to schooling may cause educational retardation. However, with appropriate management, these can be reduced. Complications, such as cardiac arrhythmias, may require urgent attention. Likewise, diabetes mellitus may require rapid stabilization.

Prognosis for the child with thalassaemia major

With changes in management, the prognosis in this disease has improved markedly. Improved transfusion regimens have resulted in children being able to lead normal lives, apart from attending for the transfusion. Chelation therapy with desferrioxamine has already delayed the appearance of signs of haemosiderosis to the third decade, and the new programmes using 10–12 hours of subcutaneous infusions offer the possibility of further improvement.

PREVENTION OF THALASSAEMIA MAJOR

Screening programmes

Screening programmes are usually offered to the following groups of people:

1 The parents and their families following the birth of an affected child.

2 Pregnant women of appropriate racial groups, followed by studies of the husbands of those who are identified as heterozygotes.

3 Couples of child-bearing age of appropriate racial groups. The screening must be voluntary and be accompanied by interviews to educate and counsel the couples.

Each of the thalassaemias is found in high frequency in specific populations, but there is sufficient overlap so that screening programmes should be designed to detect the whole variety of thalassaemias. Fig. 13.2 shows a suggested plan. Note that, in rare cases, microcytosis may be present with normal HbA_2 and HbF levels and the individual still have β- thalassaemia trait. Even more rarely, a true 'silent carrier' for β-thalassaemia trait may occur, in whom MCV, HbA_2 and HbF are all normal. Family studies often help to clarify the diagnosis. Globin chain synthesis studies are not part of a screening programme, although may be employed in specific unusual cases.

Prenatal diagnosis

The availability of this technique and what is involved should be discussed with these families as an option. Counselling in this area should lead individuals and couples to decisions and actions with which they are prepared to live. It is important that such counselling should be private and non-directive.

INVESTIGATION OF FAMILY MEMBERS

It is important that this be offered, as once an understanding of the inherited patterns of this disorder is obtained, further anxiety may arise in family members. Opportunities should therefore be made for screening and counselling of these people.

PREREQUISITES

Prerequisites for prenatal diagnosis of any disorder:

1 Acquisition of appropriate fetal tissue for study.

2 Development of assays which can use small samples.

3 Clear definition (during fetal development) of the affected individual from carriers and normals.

Prenatal diagnosis of thalassaemia is now possible due to recent developments in molecular biology and biochemistry, combined with techniques for obtaining samples of fetal amniotic fibroblasts or fetal blood. As shown in Fig. 13.1, small amounts of β chains are present in the first and second trimesters of pregnancy.

Current treatment for transfusion-dependent β-thalassaemia major is both complicated and expensive and, in addition, is not available on a worldwide basis. β-Thalassaemia is a major burden on health care systems in Italy, Greece, Turkey, Arab countries, Iran, Iraq, India, Pakistan, Thailand, Burma and Malaysia. The significant morbidity and mortality seen with the major form of the disease in these countries gives prenatal diagnosis a definite role. It is also important that families in more affluent countries be offered this option.

METHODS

There are two main approaches to the prenatal detection of haemoglobin disorders: (1) using fetal blood and (2) using fetal amniotic fibroblasts.

Prenatal diagnosis using fetal blood This approach can be used for both β and α chain disorders, and can identify mutant as well as thalassaemic conditions. Most types of β-thalassaemia cannot yet be detected in any other way.

Fetal blood sampling is done in the second trimester when the placenta is sufficiently thick and the fetal vessels sufficiently large, that a sample of pure fetal blood may be obtained. Since β chain synthesis increases during gestation, studies done as late as possible will maximize the amount of β chain synthesis which can be expected.

Fetal blood can be obtained by fetoscopy or placental aspiration with local anaesthesia. Ultrasound is used to localize the placenta, determine the gestation of the fetus and, in many cases, to guide the procedure. For fetoscopy, a Dyonics Fiberoptic Needlescope is used in a cannula, which is 2.7 mm in its largest dimension. The fetus can be inspected under direct vision and a fetal blood vessel identified in the umbilical cord near its insertion into the chorionic plate. A venepuncture is done with a 27 gauge needle which goes through a side-arm in the cannula of the fetoscope. Only 10–50 μl of fetal blood are needed and are usually drawn into a syringe along with amniotic fluid. The fetal vessel stops bleeding within a few seconds. Fetal blood loss rarely approaches 10% of blood volume. Although fetoscopy is simplified if the placenta is posterior, it can also be used in cases with anterior placentas.

Placental aspiration does not require specialized equipment, except for ultrasound. A long 20 gauge needle is advanced into the amniotic cavity and then used to gently prick the placental surface and obtain tiny samples of blood. This method has been used for anterior and posterior placentas.

Evaluation of the quality of samples obtained by fetoscopy or placental aspiration, should be performed rapidly. A particle size analyser can be used in the operating room and gives results in seconds. Fetal erythrocytes are much larger (MCV $\sim$ 140 μm^3) than those of adults (MCV $\sim$ 85 μm^3), particularly adults with thalassaemia trait (MCV $\sim$ 70μm^3). Samples with at least 5–10% fetal cells can be detected with this instrument. The precise proportion of fetal cells in the blood sample can be determined later using the acid elution method of Kleihauer and Betke.

Fetal losses have occurred, with both placental aspiration and fetoscopy being more common with the former. The incidence of fetal loss has diminished from about 15% to 5%.

Once fetal blood is obtained, cell counts are done and the samples incubated with ^{3}H-leucine, to label newly synthesized globin chains. An identical sample of maternal blood is also incubated. The cells are then lysed, globin is prepared by acid-acetone precipitation and the globin chains separated by chromatography on carboxymethyl cellulose columns in urea.

The radioactivity is determined in each of the globin peaks (γ, β and α) and the β/γ synthetic ratio is calculated.

Samples which contain a mixture of fetal and maternal blood may not lead to clearcut results unless additional steps are taken which include selective destruction of maternal red cells by specific antibodies or by selective haemolysis.

Normal β/γ ratio has a mean value of 0.1; in heterozygous thalassaemia, the mean ratio is 0.06; in homozygotes, there appear to be two groups — either there is no β chain synthesis or the ratio is below 0.025.

Prenatal diagnosis using fetal amniotic fibroblasts Disorders due to gene deletion or associated with specific abnormal genetic material, can be diagnosed by examination of fibroblast DNA. The conditions in which gene deletion is known to occur are α-thalassaemia, δβ-thalassaemia and some cases of β^{o}-thalassaemia. These disease states can be detected by molecular hybridization in solution or by gene mapping with restriction enzymes. The details of the methodology are outside the scope of this text.

Chapter 14
The Thalassaemia-like Disorders and Sickle Cell Disease

THALASSAEMIA-LIKE DISORDERS

HAEMOGLOBIN LEPORE

Hb Lepore is seen in Eastern Mediterraneans, Afro-Americans, Jamaicans and Indians.

Genetic defect

In this condition, an abnormal globin chain is present and appears to be a hybrid chain, having the *N*-terminal amino acid sequence of the normal delta chain and the carboxy-terminal amino acid sequence of the normal β chain. This defect seems to have resulted from a crossover of the adjacent delta and β loci at meiosis. The point of crossover seems to vary in different types of Hb Lepore. The nucleotide sequence of the β and γ genes is similar and this leads to their apposition during meiosis with subsequent crossover.

Pathogenesis

The Hb Lepore resembles β-thalassaemia because there is a marked decrease in synthesis of the gene product and, presumably, absence of the normal β chain locus on the affected chromosome. This is confirmed by the total absence of normal HbA and HbA_2 in patients homozygous for Hb Lepore. In the heterozygote, Hb Lepore accounts for approximately 6–15% of the total haemoglobin. It is detected by electrophoresis and has approximately the same mobility as HbS. HbA is usually low or normal, while HbF is slightly elevated.

In heterozygotes, peripheral blood findings are similar to heterozygous high A_2-β-thalassaemia. Homozygous Hb Lepore and the combination of heterozygous high A_2-β-thalassaemia with Hb Lepore are clinically indistinguishable from ordinary homozygous β-thalassaemia.

HAEMOGLOBIN CONSTANT SPRING (HbCS)

This condition has been described in association with HbH disease. In the heterozygous state, it resembles the silent carrier state of α-thalassaemia. In

HbCS, an abnormal α globin chain is synthesized, which is elongated by an additional 31 amino acids at its carboxy-terminal end. This is due to a single base mutation in the normal termination codon for α chains. As a result, the genetic code continues to read for a further 93 nucleotide residues (i.e. 31 amino acids) until the next termination codon is reached.

This abnormal haemoglobin has been found in patients of Greek, Thai and Chinese origin.

HbE-β-THALASSAEMIA

This is a common disease in Thailand. Clinically, the disease is almost as severe as homozygous β-thalassaemia. Haemoglobin electrophoresis shows HbE, HbF of approximately 50% and no HbA. It appears that when a beta thalassaemia gene is present in trans, the β^E gene is unable to compensate. This is in contrast to β^A gene and other β structural variants such as β^S and β^C.

SICKLE CELL SYNDROMES

SICKLE CELL-β-THALASSAEMIA (S-THALASSAEMIA)

This disease primarily affects people of African, Italian and Greek ancestry. Clinically, the disease resembles sickle cell disease, but usually tends to run a milder course. Splenomegaly is a common feature. Occasionally, the disease is extremely mild and the diagnosis may be made as an incidental finding.

In the peripheral blood, there is targetting, microcytosis and hypochromia of the red cells, with a variable degree of anaemia. Sickle forms of the red cells may be observed in severe cases. Hb electrophoresis reveals HbS of 60–90%, HbA of 0–30% and HbF of 1–20%. The clinical severity of the disease does not correlate well with HbA levels. HbA_2 level is often increased in S-thalassaemia.

SICKLE CELL-α-THALASSAEMIA

The presence of an alpha thalassaemia gene results in the percentage of HbS being somewhat lower than in sickle trait. Hypochromia and microcytosis are present. The clinical sequelae of S-α-thalassaemia are minimal.

SICKLE CELL ANAEMIA

Incidence

The sickle gene is a common mutant in Central Africa, the Near East, the

Mediterranean and parts of India. The gene frequency usually varies directly with the incidence of falciparum malaria.

Molecular biology of sickle haemoglobin

Sickle haemoglobin has an amino acid substitution, with a valine instead of glutamic acid in the number six position on the β chain ($\beta^S = \alpha_2\beta_2$ 6 Glut → Val). The α chain is normal.

The β^S gene is capable of a wide range of synthetic rates, depending on the nature of the non-α gene in trans. In ordinary AS trait, β^S is synthesized at approximately 40% of the rate of β^A. In S-thalassaemia, β^S-synthesis (from the β^S gene) is higher than in AS trait.

Pathogenesis of sickling

Deoxygenation is responsible for the change of red cells from the normal biconcave to the sickle shape. The molecular configuration of deoxyhaemoglobin S has been shown to be a spirally arranged sequence of molecules. Six molecules of deoxyhaemoglobin S form a ring and these rings are stacked on top of each other so that the molecules are not exactly over one another but in register, thus giving a spiral structure. The tubular structure so formed is firmer than the equivalent tubular structure with deoxyhaemoglobin A. The tubules lie alongside each other to form the sickle cell tactoids which are visible with light microscopy and which distort red cells so that they may block small blood vessels and cause tissue infarction. A red cell which has been fully sickled for several minutes is likely to be an irreversibly sickled cell. Once irreversible sickling has occurred, the red cell tends to be destroyed.

Certain haemoglobins interact well with sickle cell haemoglobin when it forms tactoids, for example HbC, HbD Punjab, HbO Arab, while others interact poorly, for example Hb Korle Bu, HbK Woolwich. The first three haemoglobins in combination with HbS give rise to sickle cell disease, while the latter two in combination result in little or no morbidity.

Fortunately, haemoglobin F and, to some extent, haemoglobin A do not interact well with sickle cell haemoglobin, thus protecting the newborn baby with sickle cell anaemia and the adult sickle cell trait carrier respectively. The higher the level of haemoglobin F, the more benign is the clinical course of sickle cell anaemia.

The plasma of patients with sickle cell disease is somewhat more viscous than normal. This is probably due to the increased level of gammaglobulin, which occurs in most cases over the age of 4 years. With deoxygenation, viscosity increases rapidly. Most cells escape from the venous to the arterial circulation before sufficient cell deformity occurs to cause entrapment. Further slowing of the circulation, deoxygenation and sickling then occur with occlusion of vessels. Since viscosity is strongly influenced by haematocrit, the patient with sickle cell disease is partially protected from occlusive episodes by anaemia, and, conversely, occlusive phenomena are more likely to occur in regions of haemoconcentration such as the spleen.

The anaemia of sickle cell disease is largely due to the rapid destruction of red blood cells by the process of sequestration and erythrophagocytosis. This process occurs within the spleen until it is infarcted and shrunken by the sickling process and then largely in the liver and throughout the reticulo-endothelial system.

The peripheral blood of patients with sickle cell disease shows marked heterogeneity of red cells. Target cells, rare spherocytes, biconcave discs, nucleated red cells, Howell-Jolly bodies and irreversibly sickled cells are all present. The number of irreversibly sickled cells is a measure of their rate of clearance by the reticuloendothelial system and is not necessarily related to the severity of the clinical symptoms. The irreversibility of sickling of these cells is a measure of membrane damage leading to membrane rigidity.

CLINICAL SYNDROMES OF DISEASE

Sickle cell trait

CLINICAL FEATURES

Most people who are heterozygous for the β^S gene, are free of symptoms. Blood counts, red cell morphology and red cell survival are all entirely normal. Haemoglobin electrophoresis shows HbS 20–40%, the remainder are haemoglobins A and A_2. A carrier of sickle cell trait may suffer an infarctive crisis on very severe deoxygenation, but this is an extremely rare occurrence. The spleen and kidneys are the most likely sites for sickling in the carrier state.

SCREENING PROGRAMMES

Where this has been done in mass screening programmes, controversy has developed about the wisdom of such programmes. Selective screening of certain groups such as pilots for light aircraft, military recruits, blood donors and pregnant women, may be a better approach in communities where there is a high incidence of the gene.

SICKLE CELL DISEASE

Clinical features

The clinical course is characterized by a 'steady state' of chronic haemolysis. This state is interrupted by *crises* which tend to be more common in early life and become less frequent when adulthood is reached.

FACTORS RESPONSIBLE FOR PRECIPITATING CRISES

1 Infections.
2 Fever.
3 Dehydration.
4 Sudden cooling.
5 Hypoxia.
6 Acidosis.

More than one of these may be operating at any time.

TYPES OF CRISES

1 *Marrow failure* This is a common cause of crisis and may be megaloblastic, especially in pregnancy, or aplastic, commonly coinciding with an infection. The danger of an aplastic crisis is that it may be overlooked and the patient may die within a few days unless transfusion is given. Careful monitoring of the reticulocyte count will define this type of crisis.

2 *Haemolytic crisis* This is probably a rare occurrence. A rise in the 'steady state' plasma bilirubin and reticulocyte count distinguishes it from an aplastic crisis. Differentiation from hepatitis, bilirubin gallstones and G6PD deficiency is essential.

3 *Sequestration crisis* A situation where blood collects in the reticuloendothelial system, especially the liver and spleen, is peculiar to sickle cell anaemia. This dramatic crisis particularly affects young infants and results in a sudden catastrophic fall in the haemoglobin concentration level in the peripheral blood. It is the commonest cause of death in children under the age of 5 years with sickle cell disease.

4 *Infarction crisis* These crises, though the most likely to draw attention because they are usually painful, may lead to the other types of crisis being overlooked. An infarctive crisis may occur in any part of the body. Chest pain, bone pain and abdominal crisis are the usual manifestations and need to be carefully differentiated from disorders causing similar pain. In infants, the small bones of the hands and feet are the most frequent sites of infarction and may become swollen and tender (hand-foot syndrome). Characteristic radiological changes are present after a week or so.

Hyposthenuria probably occurs because of chronic sickling and slow flow in proximity to the loop of Henlé, at which point the counter current-dependent renal mechanism is particularly sensitive to the rate of blood flow. This inability of the patient to concentrate urine may lead to dehydration.

Cerebral sickling may lead to severe damage to the central nervous system.

Priapism rarely occurs in young children, but may be a problem during adolescence.

Pregnancy often results in an increase in the number of vaso-occlusive episodes and urinary tract complications.

Diagnosis

Usually, the child presents as above and the diagnosis is confirmed by the presence of (1) anaemia, (2) abnormal red cell morphology, (3) a positive sickling test with sodium metabisulphite, (4) the presence of HbS and HbF on haemoglobin electrophoresis. Studies of the parents confirm the heterozygous state in each of them. Siblings should be screened at this time.

The diagnosis can be made at birth by adaptations of agar gel electrophoresis at pH 6.2 or zonal or isofocussing electrophoretic methods for the detection of HbS.

Management

PREVENTION OF CRISES

Current therapeutic emphasis is on the maintenance of the steady state by the removal of environmental factors known to precipitate a crisis. The following protective measures are recommended:

1 Good nutrition is essential. Regular supplements of folic acid are desirable and must be considered obligatory in pregnancy.

2 Prevention of infections as much as is possible, and prompt treatment of infections if they do occur.

3 The maintenance of adequate hydration is very important, especially as the patient with sickle cell anaemia is unable to concentrate his urine adequately.

4 The prevention of vascular stasis, which may occur with tight clothing or the use of tourniquets applied during an operative procedure.

5 Avoidance of cold is especially important. With cooling, the blood flow may be impeded by vasoconstriction, thus leading to sickling. This applies not only to environmental cold, but also to having ice cold drinks.

TREATMENT OF A CRISIS

1 Most cases need to be hospitalized during a crisis.

2 The environmental temperature should be warm, but not hot enough to cause excessive sweating.

3 Most crises are precipitated by an infection. This needs to be identified and treated appropriately.

4 Analgesics need to be chosen carefully, remembering the possible coexistence of G6PD deficiency and the possibility of addiction with the need for recurrent therapy.

5 Hydration with 5% glucose at 3 ml/kg/hour has a twofold effect. The blood volume is increased and this may help to 'flush out' areas of stagnating blood. Secondly, because of the Donnan equilibrium, isotonic glucose will equilibrate with intra-erythrocytic protein and cause the red cells to swell. As sickling depends on the intra-erythrocytic concentration of sickle cell haemoglobin, such hydration of the cells will have an anti-sickling effect.

6 Oxygen therapy is only of value if pulmonary oxygenation is inadequate and the arterial PO_2 is low. In the steady state, the low oxygen affinity of sickle cell haemoglobin is beneficial because it permits tissue oxygenation to be maintained with a low haematocrit level and a corresponding low viscosity of blood.

7 The role of bicarbonate therapy is mainly to prevent acidosis, not by increasing the pH, but by increasing the alkali reserve. Bicarbonate is given during crisis, being added to the 5% glucose as 10 mEq/l along with 25 mEq sodium chloride. Some people claim a reduction in the number of infarctive crises by regular use of sodium bicarbonate (up to 20 g a day in divided doses).

8 *Transfusions* Because of the low oxygen affinity of HbS, adequate tissue oxygenation can occur with haemoglobin levels as low as 6 g/100 ml or even less. In the event of a sequestration crisis, a rapid transfusion of fresh blood may be required to maintain life. Occasionally, transfusion may rapidly relieve a painful crisis.

Occasionally, as in the extreme case of a moribund patient, exchange transfusion may be necessary and may result in a miraculous recovery. This manoeuvre requires the most careful monitoring in an intensive care unit, including neutralization of citrate by calcium and the control of pH.

SPECIAL THERAPEUTIC CONSIDERATIONS

Anaesthesia In carriers of the sickle cell trait, tourniquets must not be used. Anaesthesia without the administration of oxygen (e.g. pure nitrous oxide) should be avoided. In the patient with sickle cell disease, anaesthesia is a greater risk and care should be taken to avoid factors known to precipitate a crisis. If hypoxia is likely during an operation, a preoperative exchange transfusion is indicated.

Pregnancy Careful supervision during the pregnancy is required, and a difficult or lengthy labour must be avoided. Neonatal mortality is high in this condition.

OTHER THERAPY

Treatment with urea and cyanate, which theoretically should prevent sickling, are not considered either safe or effective enough for general use.

SOCIAL ASPECTS OF SICKLE CELL DISEASE

Periodic absence from school may lead to educational retardation and subsequent difficulty in finding work. Unskilled work often tends to be in an environment which could precipitate crises. Every effort should be made to ensure that training for suitable work is given to these patients, otherwise these young people will easily join the ranks of the permanently unemployed.

RECOMMENDED READING

ALTER B. (1979) Prenatal diagnosis of haemoglobinopathies and other haematologic diseases. *Journal of Pediatrics* **95**, 4, 501.

BRITISH MEDICAL BULLETIN (1976) Haemoglobin structure, function and synthesis. *British Medical Bulletin* **32**, 3.

Iron Metabolism and Thalassaemia (1976) Birth Defects: Original Article Series **XII**, 8. Allen R. Liss, New York. 1976.

FIRST CONFERENCE ON COOLEY'S ANAEMIA (1964) *Annals of the New York Academy of Sciences.*

HUNTSMAN R.G. & LEHMANN H. (1974) Treatment of sickle cell disease. *British Journal of Haematology* **28**, 437.

MODELL B. (1977) Total management of thalassaemia major. *Archives of the Diseases of Childhood* **52**, 6, 489.

NATHAN D. & OSKI F. (eds) (1974) *Haematology of Infancy and Childhood.* W.B. Saunders, Philadelphia.

SECOND CONFERENCE ON COOLEY'S ANAEMIA (1969) *Annals of the New York Academy of Sciences.*

THIRD CONFERENCE ON COOLEY'S ANAEMIA (1974) *Annals of the New York Academy of Sciences.*

WALLACE J. (1977) *Blood Transfusions for Clinicians.* Churchill Livingstone, Edinburgh.

WEATHERALL D.J. & CLEGG J.B. (1981) *The Thalassaemia Syndromes*, 3nd edn. Blackwell Scientific Publications, Oxford.

ZAINO E.C. & ROBERTS R. (eds) (1977) *Chelation Therapy in Chronic Iron Overload.* Symposia Specialists, Miami.

Chapter 15
Haemolytic Disease of the Newborn (HDN)

Haemolytic disease of the fetus and newborn occurs when there is the following combination of circumstances: (1) the fetus has red cell antigens which are not present on the mother's red cells; (2) the mother has circulating antibodies to these antigens; (3) the maternal antibodies can cross the placenta and cause haemolysis of fetal red cells.

The most common fetal red cell antigens which induce such antibodies are: (1) A or B antigens, as seen in ABO incompatibility; (2) Rh antigens, as seen in Rh immunization; (3) rare red cell antigens.

Although antibodies to A and B antigens are more frequently detected in maternal serum, Rh antibodies result in more frequent and more severe haemolysis of fetal red cells.

Rh HAEMOLYTIC DISEASE

Antigens

Of the Rh antigens, the most significant and clinically important is the D antigen. The presence of this antigen on the erythrocyte makes that cell 'Rh-positive' and its absence, referred to in notational form as 'd', makes it 'Rh-negative'. There are two major groups of other antigens related to the D antigen and these are referred to as Cc and Ee. The three antigenic sites can be regarded as the product of a single gene. Their frequency in Caucasian populations is cDE(R^2) 14%, CDe (R^1) 41% and cde(r) 39%. As the Rh groups are coded from single genes on single chromosomes, pairing results in a prevalence of R^1R^2, i.e. homozygous Rh-positive, or Rr heterozygous Rh-positive. In 15% of the population, pairing results in rr, i.e. Rh-negative. The composition of the three antigens in both *cis* and *trans* affects the relative reactivity of the D antigen.

While 15% of pregnant women are Rh-negative, only approximately 9% will carry an Rh-positive fetus. The incidence of haemolytic disease in these pregnancies at risk is 7%.

Antibodies

Anti-D antibodies are by far the most important, however haemolytic disease may also occur with anti-c and anti-E antibodies. Rh antibodies are primarily immunoglobulins of the IgM or IgG type. IgM are the first to appear, but as they do not cross the placenta, they play no part in the pathogenesis of haemolytic disease. Only IgG antibodies cross the placenta. Both IgM and IgG antibodies may be detected in maternal serum, the former as complete (or 'saline') antibodies, the latter as incomplete antibodies whose presence is revealed only after reaction of the sensitized cells with anti-human IgG antibody (i.e. a Coombs' reaction) or after suspension in albumin, or treatment with enzymes such as papain. It is the level of IgG anti-D antibodies which is of clinical importance.

The interaction of anti-D with a D-positive erythrocyte does not result in activation of the complement system. The rate of entry of IgG into the fetal circulation is slow. This may account for the milder disease in some first affected children. Subsequent children are more severely affected, and the severity appears to be more uniform in later pregnancies.

Pathogenesis

IMMUNIZATION OF THE MOTHER

Fetal erythrocytes cross the placenta to enter the maternal circulation. Repeated injections of small quantities of red cells increase the likelihood of immunization, but not all women will develop antibodies. Primary immunization with the appearance of anti-D antibodies may not be evident for several months after the primary stimulus. A second injection of cells in an immunized subject results in a rapid rise in antibody levels.

Fetal erythrocytes can be found in the maternal circulation as early as the second month of pregnancy, especially if the pregnancy is complicated by such events as threatened abortion. The volume of cells is usually about 0.05–0.1 ml. Rh immunization may occur at any time during pregnancy, but is more likely if the pregnancy is complicated by toxaemia, antepartum haemorrhage, Caesarean section or manual removal of the placenta. However, normal delivery, ectopic pregnancy or therapeutic abortion can also result in Rh immunization. Although fetal red cells may be detected in the maternal circulation using the acid elution test of Kleihauer-Betke, not all mothers produce detectable antibodies. Where there is also ABO incompatibility, the fetal red cells may be destroyed before stimulating Rh antibody production. To summarize, of the group of Rh-negative women at risk of developing Rh antibodies, 0.1% develop weak antibodies by the end of their first pregnancy with an Rh-positive fetus; 7.5% develop antibodies in the first 6 months after delivery; and a further 7.5% do not develop antibodies until their next pregnancy with an Rh-positive fetus.

Blood transfusion with Rh incompatible blood is nowadays an uncommon cause of Rh immunization.

DESTRUCTION OF FETAL ERYTHROCYTES

The transfer of anti-D antibody into the fetal circulation and the subsequent destruction of Rh-positive fetal erythrocytes represents the basic pathogenic mechanism responsible for haemolytic disease of the newborn. The rate of splenic destruction of IgG sensitized erythrocytes (i.e. extravascular haemolysis) depends on the capacity of the reticuloendothelial system to destroy these cells. The erythrocytes are ingested by macrophages in the spleen and digested by lysosomal proteolytic enzymes and haem oxygenase, resulting in the production of ferritin, bilirubin and carbon monoxide. With large amounts of anti-D on the erythrocytes, intravascular haemolysis may also occur, resulting in elevated levels of plasma haemoglobin and methaemalbumin.

RESPONSE OF THE FETUS TO ERYTHROCYTE DESTRUCTION

The anaemia resulting from erythrocyte destruction leads to increased production of erythropoietin in the fetus and increased red cell production. Erythropoietic tissue increases in the marrow as well as in the liver and spleen, contributing to their enlargement. Numerous normoblasts and reticulocytes are seen in the peripheral blood. In severe Rh disease, increased erythropoiesis is unable to compensate for the anaemia; the plasma volume increases; cardiac failure develops followed by tissue hypoxia, metabolic acidosis and death.

The characteristic syndrome of massive oedema, ascites and very severe haemolytic disease is known as hydrops fetalis. The accumulation of fluid is thought to be due to a combination of cardiac failure, raised venous pressure associated with fetal asphyxia and a fall in osmotic pressure in part due to a fall in the serum proteins. Oedema of the chorionic villi of the placenta may also contribute by interfering with water transport across the villi.

Hyperplasia of the β cells of the pancreas also occurs with increased insulin production and postnatal hypoglycaemia. In the liver, focal cellular necrosis may occur, resulting in high levels of direct bilirubin at birth and prolonged obstructive jaundice in the neonate.

At the other end of the spectrum, haemolysis may be mild with minimal anaemia and evidence of extramedullary erythropoiesis at birth.

BILIRUBIN METABOLISM

As mentioned earlier, antibody coated red cells in the spleen are ingested by macrophages and digested to produce bilirubin. This bilirubin is lipid soluble and, therefore, can cross the cell membrane and enter the plasma where it binds to plasma albumin. Any unbound bilirubin accumulates as free bilirubin and it is this form which is toxic to the nervous system.

In the fetus, bilirubin levels are not high as the placenta can freely transport unconjugated bilirubin as a lipid soluble material. The bilirubin then binds to maternal albumin. Small quantities of bilirubin enter amniotic fluid and this phenomenon serves as the basis for the antepartum diagnostic tests of the severity of haemolysis using amniocentesis to determine bilirubin levels (see Fig. 15.1).

Factors influencing albumin-bilirubin binding in the neonate

1 *Serum albumin level* Both prematurity and Rh disease are associated with hypoalbuminaemia.

2 *Acidosis* The binding by albumin of free bilirubin diminishes with falling pH.

3 *Competition for binding sites* Both naturally occurring substances and medications compete with bilirubin for the same binding sites on albumin. If

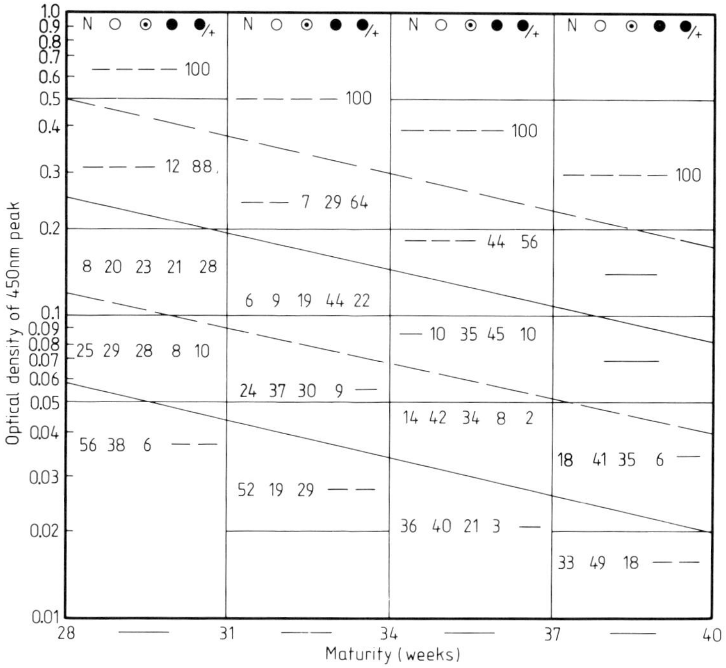

Fig. 15.1 Liley's three zone chart for estimating the severity of haemolytic disease of the newborn. The optical density of the 450 nm peak is plotted against maturity of the fetus. For each gestational period and for each 450 nm reading are shown the probabilities of the severity of haemolytic disease from the intra-uterine death; varying degrees of anaemia (Hb in g/100ml) or an unaffected fetus. ○: ≥14; ⊙: 11–13.9; ●: 8–10.9; ●/+: ≤7.9, intra-uterine death; N: unaffected. Thus in the gestation period of 28–31 weeks, an optical density reading of 0.4 at the 450 nm peak indicates an 88% probability of intra-uterine death or a Hb < 7.9 g% at birth and a 12% probability of Hb 8–10 g% at time of birth. On the other hand, an optical density reading of 0.04 indicates a 56% chance of an unaffected pregnancy; 38% chance of Hb 14 g% or more at birth and a 6% chance of a Hb of 11–13.9 g% at birth. (Compiled from data obtained at the Queen Victoria Medical Centre, Melbourne, and presented to the authors by courtesy of Dr J. Campbell.)

binding sites are occupied by the following, then less free bilirubin can be bound:
(a) free fatty acids — likely to be present in ill, fasting infants.
(b) haematin — likely to be present in the plasma of Rh affected infants.
(c) salicylates, sulphonamides, novobiocin and benzoate (as in valium).
(d) possibly ampicillin and gentamicin.

After birth, bilirubin bound to albumin is taken up by the liver. Bilirubin enters the hepatic cell in the free form and is quickly bound to binding proteins. It is then conjugated as a bilirubin glucuronide by means of the enzyme, glucuronyl transferase, which is markedly deficient in the newborn. Conjugated bilirubin is water soluble and is excreted in the bile and urine. A small amount of bilirubin is also lost through the wall of the intestine, and some is broken down into water soluble products. Exposure to light increases these water soluble products and this is the basis of phototherapy. These water soluble products are also excreted in the bile and urine, and there is no evidence to suggest that they, in themselves, are toxic.

BILIRUBIN ENCEPHALOPATHY

The neurological damage from bilirubin may result in death or severe brain damage. At post-mortem, the basal ganglia and cerebellum show yellow staining, i.e. kernicterus. Minor neurological defects such as high frequency nerve deafness, behaviour and learning disorders may occur. The bilirubin-albumin complex cannot cross the intact blood-brain barrier to cause neurological damage. However, both hypoxia and severe hypoglycaemia may increase the permeability of the blood-brain barrier to bilirubin.

From the above, it can be seen that it is not the absolute level of serum bilirubin that determines the risk of bilirubin encephalopathy, but the degree to which the albumin binding sites are occupied and the permeability of the blood-brain barrier. A healthy baby, with normal serum albumin, who has not sustained acidosis, hypoxia or hypoglycaemia, may be at no risk with a very high serum bilirubin; on the other hand, an ill, premature or hydropic infant, with low serum albumin, hypoxia, acidosis and hypoglycaemia, may be at risk from a quite low level. The ideal laboratory test, which measures the availability of albumin-bilirubin binding sites, has not as yet been coordinated with clinical outcome.

Management

PREVENTION OF Rh IMMUNIZATION IN THE MOTHER AT RISK

The use of intramuscular human anti-D gammaglobulin (300 μg) has dramatically reduced the incidence of Rh immunization in pregnancy. Anti-D should be administered following threatened or therapeutic abortion and ectopic pregnancy in all Rh-negative women within 72 hours of any form of delivery of an Rh-positive infant. Administration of blood products (e.g. platelets) which come fom an Rh-postive donor, when administered to an Rh-negative female, should be accompanied by an anti-D injection. Although platelets do not carry the D antigen, there may be sufficient red cell contamination of the platelets to immunize the recipient.

PREVENTION OF INTRAUTERINE DEATH

Early identification of Rh-negative patients who have been sensitized by Rh-positive cells, is essential. Preferably, detailed Rh typing should be performed at the first antenatal visit. However, in most cases, routine testing is limited to the D antigen. Consequently, unexpected haemolytic disease of the newborn may arise from incompatibility of rare antigens in occasional Rh-positive women.

When Rh antibodies are not evident at the first visit, the screening should be repeated at 28 weeks and 36 weeks gestation, as antibodies may appear during the pregnancy. The level of such antibodies will give an indication of the risk to the fetus of haemolytic disease and provide guidance to the obstetrician for the subsequent management of the pregnancy.

As mentioned, amniocentesis can be performed to determine the severity of disease in an affected fetus. The procedure is undertaken only in pregnancies where the antibody titre is of such a level as to indicate moderate or severe disease, or in women who have a past history of erythroblastosis. The timing of this procedure may need to be as early as 20 weeks gestation when severe disease is anticipated but, in moderately severe disease, the procedure is usually performed at 28–30 weeks of gestation. In performing amniocentesis, the placenta is localized using sonography and, if possible, avoided, as puncture could lead to massive immunization of the mother. The degree of disease in the fetus is assessed by measuring the optical density of the amniotic fluid using spectrophotometric methods. The optical density at the 450 nm peak ($\Delta\ OD_{450}$) is plotted on Liley's three zone chart (Fig. 15.1). The interpretation of Fig. 15.1 is outlined in the legend.

Amniocentesis may need to be repeated at weekly intervals if the $\Delta\ OD_{450}$ is in the danger zones, or after a 3–4 week interval if the $\Delta\ OD_{450}$ is very low.

When careful consideration of analyses of amniotic fluid indicates serious fetal haemolytic disease, intrauterine transfusion may be life saving. Intrauterine transfusion is rarely initiated before 23 weeks gestation. The earlier this procedure is initiated, the worse the prognosis. Under sonographic and, in some cases, fluoroscopic control, Rh-negative low titre anti-A and anti-B haemolysin packed red cells are introduced into the fetal peritoneal cavity by means of a needle or catheter. In severely affected fetuses, the salvage rate is 30–40%. The risk to the mother is minimal. The high risk infant may require several intrauterine transfusions and this may induce premature delivery. In any case, in these severely affected infants, delivery before 34 weeks gestation is desirable. In the less severely affected infant, induction of labour and delivery are usually required before term to avoid stillbirth.

POSTNATAL MANAGEMENT

As most babies with haemolytic disease are identified during antenatal assessment and delivered by early induction of labour, it is possible to have skilled obstetric and neonatal staff present at the time of delivery. The most common problems encountered in the neonate are prematurity, anaemia and asphyxia.

Initial efforts are usually directed towards effective resuscitation, establishing an optimal environment, minimizing oxygen consumption by stabilizing body temperature, monitoring and stabilizing blood pressure, and correcting acidosis and hypoglycaemia. Immediate exchange transfusion is occasionally necessary, but usually reserved for the neonate with severely compromised respiratory function or asphyxia at birth in association with severe anaemia. In such an infant, a limited exchange transfusion using packed red cells (O Rh-negative with low titres of anti-A and anti-B haemolysins) in sufficient amount to correct the anaemia, is performed as part of the emergency resuscitation. Endotracheal intubation and ventilation may be required prior to the procedure.

Examination of cord blood confirms the diagnosis of haemolytic disease and gives some indication of its severity. However, in infants who have received intrauterine transfusions, fetal erythrocytes may be reduced or absent, the Coombs' test negative and Haemoglobin F measurement less than 2%. This is perhaps the result of suppression of fetal erythropoiesis by infused adult blood, or to continuing destruction of mature fetal cells and reticulocytes by anti-D antibody.

If immediate exchange transfusion is not indicated, levels of haemoglobin and unconjugated bilirubin in cord blood are used to predict whether

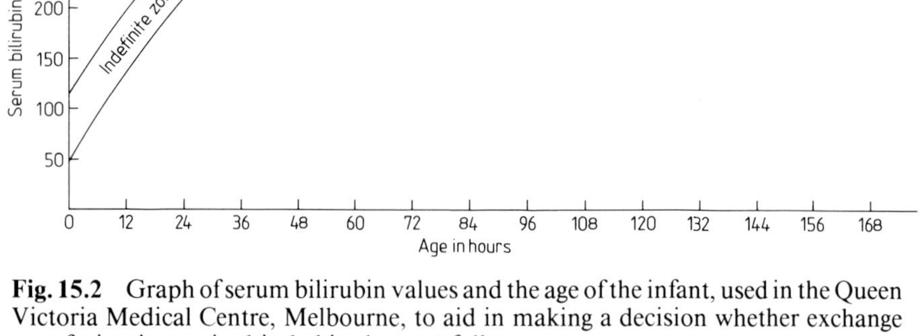

Fig. 15.2 Graph of serum bilirubin values and the age of the infant, used in the Queen Victoria Medical Centre, Melbourne, to aid in making a decision whether exchange transfusion is required in babies born at full term.

exchange transfusion in the first 6–12 hours of life is advisable. The usual criteria are a cord haemoglobin of less than 14 g/100 ml and/or cord indirect bilirubin greater than 70 μmol/l. This exchange transfusion is best performed after the infant has adjusted to extrauterine life and associated conditions such as asphyxia, respiratory distress or hypoglycaemia have been stabilized.

By means of this transfusion, anaemia is corrected and sensitized red cells, antibody and bilirubin are removed. The need for further exchange transfusions is determined by measurements of serum bilirubin at the beginning and end of each exchange transfusion, and at 6–12 hourly intervals. These values are graphed on suitable charts (Figs 15.2, 15.3). However, interpretation of these results must take into account the possible adverse effects of associated conditions such as hypoxia, acidosis and hypoglycaemia, which could necessitate exchange transfusion at a lower level of serum bilirubin than is indicated on the charts, in order to prevent bilirubin encephalopathy.

In exchange transfusions for hyperbilirubinaemia, whole blood with or without added albumin, is used in an attempt to increase the albumin-binding sites. Blood for these subsequent exchange transfusions must be compatible on crossmatch with both infant and maternal serum. Hyperkalaemia and hypernatraemia can be avoided by using blood less than 3 days old, whereas acidosis and hypocalcaemia associated with citrate anticoagulants, an extra hazard if infants are ill, can be avoided by using blood anticoagulated with heparin. The amount of blood exchanged is usually twice the infant's blood volume, and the exchange is made via the umbilical vein and/or artery. When performed by skilled operators, complications are rare.

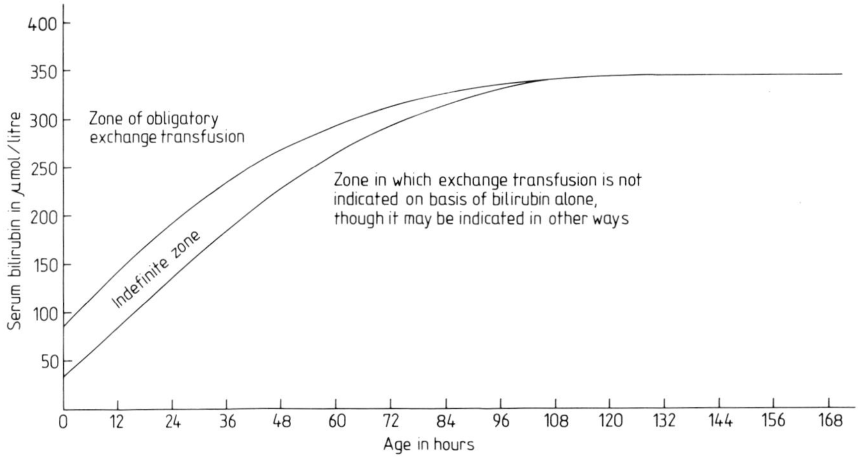

Fig. 15.3 Graph of serum bilirubin values and the age of the infant, used in the Queen Victoria Medical Centre, Melbourne, to aid in making a decision whether exchange transfusion is required in premature babies.

Phototherapy has no place in the early treatment of haemolytic disease of the newborn, especially when haemolysis is severe and rapid. After two or three days, it may be helpful in delaying the rise in serum bilirubin levels. A light source of 450 wavelength is used. When it is used, care must be taken that anaemia or hyperbilirubinaemia are not missed and that the procedure does not induce dehydration.

Elevated levels of direct bilirubin as a result of obstructive jaundice are common in severe haemolytic disease, but usually clear spontaneously.

Thrombocytopenia may occur, especially after several exchange transfusions and may require platelet infusions, as the risk of intracranial haemorrhage is high in these infants. Disseminated intravascular coagulation should be considered in the thrombocytopenic infant, but is rarely present.

'Late' anaemia is most likely to occur in the mildly affected infant who has not required exchange transfusion, but may also occur in exchange transfused infants, especially if measureable Rh antibody persists for several weeks.

Prognosis

The major risks to the fetus and infant are intrauterine death, severe neonatal anaemia and hyperbilirubinaemia. These problems can in most cases be overcome with appropriate management. However, there are many possibilities for errors of judgement as well as the hazards of intrauterine transfusion, exchange transfusion and phototherapy. When such pregnancies are managed by teams of obstetricians, paediatricians and haematologists who are experienced in treating this disorder, there are few sequelae in babies who manage to survive intrauterine life.

ABO HAEMOLYTIC DISEASE

This disease is limited to mothers of blood group O and affects infants of blood group A or B. Anti-A and anti-B antibodies develop early in life and result from immune stimulation by the A or B substance contained in food and bacteria. The antibody levels may increase with age. They are found in the IgA, IgM and IgG fractions of immunoglobulins, but only the IgG fraction can cross the placenta and cause haemolysis of fetal red cells.

About 15% of all pregnancies are ABO incompatible. However, actual haemolytic disease of the newborn only occurs in about 3%. The disease, although much more common (approximately five times) than Rh incompatibility, is relatively mild in its clinical course.

Diagnosis

1 Appropriate blood groups in the mother and baby.

2 The red blood cell of the newborn has a much lower content of A or B reactive sites than that seen in the adult. This explains the weekly reactive Coombs' test in ABO haemolytic disease.

3 Antibody eluted from these cells reacts strongly with adult group A erythrocytes.

Pathogenesis

The disease appears to be due to the entrance of maternal IgG anti-A (or -B) into the fetal circulation and its reaction with fetal erythrocytes. The degree of interaction is determined by the A antigen strength on the erythrocyte. It is probably modified by the presence of soluble A or B substance in the plasma of these infants. This possibility is supported by the observation that anti-A and anti-B antibodies disappear from the circulation of the newborn in the first three days of life.

Red cell destruction can occur by either intravascular or extravascular haemolysis, but appears to result primarily from extravascular haemolysis.

Clinical features

The first sign is usually rapidly developing jaundice in the first 24 hours of life: splenomegaly is unusual. Anaemia is mild or absent. The blood film shows spherocytes and occasional erythroblasts.

Management

Adequate warmth, fluids and early feeding will help to minimize the severity of jaundice. Early introduction of phototherapy reduces the need for exchange transfusion. Serum bilirubin should be measured and graphed at 12 hourly intervals until sustained falls occur. Exchange transfusion is occasionally required (see Figs 15.2, 15.3).

Prognosis

With adequate management of the hyperbilirubinaemia, there are no sequelae.

HAEMOLYTIC DISEASE DUE TO RARE RED CELL ANTIGENS

The majority of these are caused by anti-Kell and anti-Duffy antibodies. The infrequency of disease in this group is due to the relatively low potency of these antigens.

The diagnosis and therapy of these diseases are identical to those of Rh haemolytic disease of the newborn.

RECOMMENDED READING

MAISLES M.J. (1975) Neonatal jaundice and phototherapy. *Neonatology: Pathophysiology and Management of the Newborn* (ed. G.P. AVERY), p.354. W.B. Saunders, Philadelphia.

OSKI F. & NAIMAN J. (1972) *Haematologic Problems in Newborn*, 2nd edn, p.176. W.B. SAUNDERS, Philadelphia.

OSKI F. (1975) Haematological problems. *Neonatology: Pathophysiology and Management of the Newborn* (ed. G.B. AVERY), p.385. W. B. Saunders, Philadelphia.

Chapter 16
Solid Tumours

The disciplines of haematology and oncology are united in one department in the majority of children's hospitals and paediatric divisions of cancer treatment centres. For the sake of convenience, the chapters on solid tumours have been gathered together at the end of this book, but to emphasize the unity of haematology and oncology in paediatrics, that on the leukaemias has been placed with the chapters on disorders of white cells. This chapter outlines the principles of management and some details of clinical features, differential diagnosis and therapeutic approaches in the more common paediatric solid tumours. The text is a practical outline rather than a complete description of paediatric oncology, which can be found in the specialized text books.

The field of paediatric oncology is rapidly changing and there are still many therapeutic strategies which are a matter of opinion and experience rather than established by experimental evidence. Factual knowledge on the intensity and duration of treatment has yet to be established by randomized clinical trials in most tumours and it is likely that, in the future, some of the treatment programmes outlined in the chapters that follow may prove to be incorrect. New methods of investigation may also supersede the more conventional ones outlined in the text. Development of monoclonal antibodies to paediatric tumours and recombinant DNA techniques for diagnosis and definition of aetiology may dramatically alter management of solid tumours.

Despite these exciting new developments and the many uncertainties, there is a need to define and describe a core of knowledge that can be applied to patients whose needs have to be met now, rather than in the future.

It must be remembered when considering the treatment and investigative modalities currently available, that they have long-term undesirable effects in the child who is a growing and evolving organism. The aim of treatment is to achieve a genuine cure with minimal long-term morbidity. The treatment of childhood cancer remains a trade-off between a fatal disease and potential toxicity. The paediatric haematologist/oncologist has a special duty to consider long-term effects of treatment and to attempt to design therapeutic regimens which can be justified by a minimum rate of long-term complications, but which maximize the chance of cure from the malignancy. We must avoid, if at all possible, treatment regimens which result in bone deformity and major reduction of stature. We should try and select therapeutic regimens which, on the basis of current knowledge, are effective and least oncogenic. We must be aware of the potential for endocrinologic toxicity and interference with fertility.

Children with tumours often undergo emotional trauma related to the consequences of treatment and the effects of the disease on the family. The paediatric haematologist/oncologist can play an active role in alleviating some of these stresses by sympathetic support of the patient and the family, by attention to their emotional and social needs and by imparting information which is accurate and tailored to the needs of the particular family. The haematologist/oncologist should not transmit to their patient and family their own anxieties and their still all too frequent sense of defeat. The outline of the approach to the families of children with malignancy and the management of the dying child are discussed in the chapter on leukaemia (Chapter 7).

Incidence

Solid tumours account for approximately two-thirds of cases of malignancy in children. Of these, primary central nervous system tumours are the commonest, accounting for nearly 20% of malignant disease of childhood. Malignant lymphomas, neuroblastoma and Wilms' tumour all occur with approximately equal frequency. The frequency of soft tissue and bone sarcomas, as well as retinoblastoma, is low (Table 16.1).

The improved results in childhood cancer are in large part due to the introduction of a multidisciplinary approach to treatment as exemplified by the tumour board or combined therapy clinic. This combined approach advises on the correct use of diagnostic procedures and definitive therapy involving the disciplines of surgery, radiation therapy and chemotherapy. If a multidisciplinary team is not available at a particular centre, then the patient should be referred to a unit where such an approach is practised. It is only by this means that the most effective treatment can be given. Usually, the medical oncologist is the person who should lead the team and act as the primary physician.

Diagnosis and staging

The key to optimal treatment of solid tumours is to establish an accurate

Table 16.1 Incidence of specific types of cancer in children.

Type of cancer	Frequency (%)
Leukaemia	36
Lymphoma–Hodgkin's disease	7
CNS tumours	19
Neuroblastoma	9
Wilms' tumour	8
Sarcomas (bone and soft tissue)	8

pathological diagnosis and to accurately stage the tumour. The prognosis and the intensity and nature of treatment are determined by the stage of the tumour.

Once the clinical differential diagnosis has been established, the appropriate diagnostic and staging procedures can be undertaken. Prior to surgery, a full blood examination and platelet count and chest X-ray are usually obtained. Further radiology such as intravenous pyelography may help differentiate between renal and extra renal lesions. Neuroradiologic studies are necessary in the case of a suspected primary CNS tumour. Radionucleotide studies and computerized axial tomography (CAT) have supplanted invasive radiological techniques, such as angiography, in most institutions. By these means, the stage of the tumour may be established before biopsy or excision is performed. Whenever possible, the presence of tumour markers should be sought. These include plasma levels of catecholamines and other products of noradrenaline metabolism, α-fetoproteins, or carcinoembryonic antigen. In many instances, final staging will depend upon the surgeon's findings at operation and precise assessment by the surgeon of the extent of the tumour and biopsy of appropriate lymph node groups is essential in staging.

If the clinical diagnosis is of a localized tumour, i.e. Stage I, then the surgical approach should be one of complete resection without preliminary biopsy (excisional biopsy). For example, in a patient with an abdominal mass with the characteristics of a Wilms' tumour on intravenous pyelography, the correct surgical procedure is nephrectomy without biopsy, as this avoids potential contamination of the peritoneal cavity by tumour cells. In this instance, the surgical procedure is both diagnostic and potentially curative. If generalized lymphadenopathy is present, then excisional biopsy of an involved node will be diagnostic. Further staging procedures can then be planned according to the pathological diagnosis. Incisional biopsy only is indicated when total tumour removal will lead to unacceptable physiological or functional impairment, when chemotherapy and/or radiotherapy may be equally as effective and less mutilating, or when widespread tumour excludes the possibility of total tumour excision.

The importance of an adequate biopsy cannot be overstressed. The tissues should be handled gently. Equally important is the pathological handling of the specimen, where imprints may be obtained and material sent for electron microscopy and immunological investigation before formalin fixation. Once the pathological diagnosis is established, other appropriate staging procedures which had not previously been undertaken, are performed. In general, this involves skeletal survey and/or bone scans, more extensive CAT scanning and bone marrow examination for malignant cells. In special circumstances, e.g. rhabdomyosarcoma of the head and neck and retinoblastoma, CSF examination for malignant cells is also required. For most tumours,

Stage I refers to local tumour.

Stage II to local tumour with microscopic extension to the edge of the excision.
Stage III to surgically irremovable tumours or those with regional node involvement.
Stage IV to those with general dissemination.

The staging system applied for each pathological type of tumour will be amplified in the appropriate chapters.

Principles of treatment

A curative approach should be undertaken at presentation for all children with solid tumours, even those with widespread metastatic disease at presentation. Treatment should be individualized for each particular pathological subtype of tumour. In general, surgery and adjuvant chemotherapy are used alone for most Stage I tumours as, in many instances, postoperative irradiation does not improve long-term survival and is associated with undesirable side-effects, e.g. Wilms' tumour, rhabdomyosarcoma. Surgery, chemotherapy and postoperative irradiation are required for most Stage II tumours. In Stage III tumours, chemotherapy and irradiation therapy are the mainstays of treatment. With aggressive chemotherapy and/or irradiation, some Stage III tumours can be converted to Stage I and Stage II tumours and it may be feasible to resect residual tumour bulk. Maintenance chemotherapy is continued for a variable length of time ranging from 6–24 months.

For Stage IV tumours, chemotherapy is the main method of treatment, but radiotherapy may be given to areas of bulk disease or to provide rapid relief of symptoms of obstruction. Surgical excision is rarely called for, apart from that necessary to establish the pathologic diagnosis.

RADIATION THERAPY

Ionizing radiation is a very effective way of treating the primary tumour. The sensitivity of the tumour to irradiation varies with the biological nature of the cells that compose it and, in general, is similar to that seen with chemotherapy. The limitations of irradiation are its deleterious effects on normal tissue, growth retardation and oncogenic potential. The 'therapeutic ratio' depends on the sensitivity of the tumour and the tolerance of neighbouring tissues and organs. The 'therapeutic ratio' has been increased by the use of megavoltage therapy which has a sharper beam edge, better depth penetration and hence a more homogenous dose distribution and more skin and bone sparing effects.

In planning treatment volumes, one endeavours to encompass the local extent of the tumour and allow for a margin of normal tissue. The extent of the normal margin depends on the proximity of vital organs, e.g. in the limb a margin of 5 cm of normal tissue may be reasonable, while in the pelvis a margin of 3 cm may be the maximum without causing serious damage to bladder and/or rectum. In planning treatment volumes, it is always necessary to have accurate clinical and surgical information and supplemental information with radiology, nuclear isotopes and CAT scans. In addition, knowledge of the natural history and sites of local infiltration are used to plan the field, e.g. in patients with parameningeal rhabdomyosarcoma extension of tumour to the base of the skull is sufficiently common to include it in the irradiation field.

To achieve reproducible treatment, full cooperation of the child is required. This can usually be achieved by sympathetic handling of the child, familiarization with the equipment and staff and mild sedation. In very young or severely disturbed children, light anaesthesia may be necessary to permit adequate irradiation.

Shielding of vital organs such as kidney or liver is used to prevent their damage during irradiation. When planning irradiation, the cumulative toxicity of chemotherapy and irradiation must be taken into account. Of particular danger are the cumulative toxicity of irradiation and cyclophosphamide on the bladder, irradiation and adriamycin on heart and oesophagus, irradiation and actinomycin D on liver, irradiation and actinomycin D on skin and mucous membranes, and the potential for leucoencephalopathy of CNS irradiation and systemic methotrexate or intrathecal methotrexate when there is interference with CSF circulation. For all these reasons, it is essential that the radiotherapist be a member of the medical and allied professions team undertaking the management of paediatric malignancies.

ADJUVANT CHEMOTHERAPY

Adjuvant chemotherapy plays a key role in the treatment of childhood solid tumours, being, to a major degree, responsible for both the significant increase in survival time and the percentage cured. The optimal role of chemotherapy in patients with primary CNS tumours has yet to be established. Because of the potential toxicity of many cancer chemotherapeutic agents, they should only be administered by physicians experienced in their use and at centres where adequate support facilities are available. The specific chemotherapy for individual tumour types will be discussed in succeeding chapters.

The general principles of chemotherapy are as follows: Firstly and most importantly, chemotherapy is used curatively to suppress micrometastases and local recurrences in cases where the primary can be controlled with surgery, e.g. Wilms' tumour, rhabdomyosarcoma, osteosarcoma or with irradiation, e.g. Ewing's sarcoma. Secondly and again curatively, to reduce the size of a massive tumour (often in conjunction with irradiation therapy), thus making it surgically resectable, e.g. rhabdomyosarcoma of the pelvis. Thirdly, in patients with metastatic disease to obtain a remission (again, often in conjunction with irradiation to the primary lesion or areas of bulk disease) and to maintain this remission or permit effective alternative means of consolidation of remission, as in neuroblastoma and lymphoma.

Table 16.2 Anti-cancer drugs: class, mode of action, toxicity.

Drug	Route	Toxicity	Major site of action in cell cycle	Major use	Minor use
Alkylating agents					
Nitrogen mustard (Mustine)	i.v.	Myelosuppression Nausea and vomiting Alopecia Local irritant	Cycle specific	Lymphomas	Histiocytosis X Neuroblastoma Wilms' tumour
Cyclophosphamide (Cytoxan, Endoxan)	i.v, i.m. oral	Myelosuppression Nausea and vomiting Alopecia Haemorrhagic cystitis Immunosuppression	Cycle specific	Lymphoma ALL Neuroblastoma Rhabdomyosarcoma Ewing's sarcoma	Osteosarcoma Wilms' tumour Retinoblastoma
Chlorambucil (Leukeran)	oral	Myelosuppression Hepatotoxicity	Cycle specific	Lymphoma Histiocytosis X Chronic lymphatic leukaemia	Ovarian cancer
Busulphan (Myleran)	oral	Myelosuppression Nausea and vomiting Alopecia Interstitial pulmonary fibrosis	Cycle specific	Chronic myeloid leukaemia	
Dimethyl imidazole carboxamide (DIC)	i.v.	Myelosuppression Pain on infusion	Cycle specific	Ewing's sarcoma Soft tissue sarcoma Neuroblastoma	

M

Drug	Route	Toxicity	Major site of action in cell cycle	Major use	Minor use
Antimetabolites					
Methotrexate (Aminopterin)	oral i.v., i.m., i.t.	Mucosal Myelosuppression Hepatic Renal Osteoporosis	Phase specific	Acute lymphatic leukaemia Choriocarcinoma Lymphoma Osteosarcoma	Testicular tumours Teratoma
6-Mercaptopurine (Purinethol)	oral	Myelosuppression Hepatic Immunosuppression	Phase specific	Acute leukaemia	
Cytosine arabinoside (Cytosar) (Cytarabine) (Ara-C)	i.v., i.m., subcutaneous i.t.	Myelosuppression Hepatic Nausea and vomiting	Phase specific	Acute leukaemia Lymphoma CNS leukaemia	
Fluorouracil (5-FU)	i.v. oral	Mucosal Nausea and vomiting Myelosuppression	Phase specific	Ewing's sarcoma Hepatoma	Carcinoma
Antibiotics					
Actinomycin D (Cosmegen)	i.v.	Myelosuppression Mucosal Local irritant Radiomimetic	Cycle specific	Wilms' tumour Choriocarcinoma Testicular tumour Ewing's sarcoma	Soft tissue sarcoma Neuroblastoma
Daunorubicin (Daunomycin) (Rubidomycin) (Cerubidin)	i.v.	Myelosuppression Nausea and vomiting Alopecia Cardiac (total dose related)	Cycle specific	Acute leukaemia	Neuroblastoma

Table 16.2 Anti-cancer drugs: class, mode of action, toxicity (continued).

Drug	Route	Toxicity	Major site of action in cell cycle	Major use	Minor use
Adriamycin (Doxorubicin)	i.v.	Myelosuppression Nausea and vomiting Mucosal Local irritant Cardiac (total dose related)	Cycle specific	Acute leukaemia Osteosarcoma Ewing's sarcoma Neuroblastoma Rhabdomyosarcoma Lymphoma	Wilms' tumour
Bleomycin (Blenoxane)	i.v., i.m., subcutaneous	Pulmonary Skin Hypotension Fever	Cycle specific	Lymphoma	Osteosarcoma
Plant alkaloids					
Vincristine (Oncovin)	i.v.	Peripheral neuropathy Abdominal pain Myelosuppression Local irritant Alopecia	Phase specific	Acute leukaemia Wilms' tumour Rhabdomyosarcoma Ewing's sarcoma Lymphoma Neuroblastoma	Histiocytosis X CNS tumours Retinoblastoma
Vinblastine (Velban)	i.v.	Myelosuppression Alopecia Local irritant	Phase specific	Histiocytosis X Lymphoma	Testicular tumours
Enzymes					
E. coli asparaginase Erwinia caratovora asparaginase	i.v., i.m.	Anaphylactic reaction Pancreatitis Hyperglycaemia Hepatic	Phase specific	Acute lymphatic leukaemia Lymphoma	

Drug	Route	Toxicity	Major site of action in cell cycle	Major use	Minor use
Miscellaneous					
Procarbazine (Natulan)	oral	Myelosuppression Nausea and vomiting CNS depression	Cycle specific	Hodgkin's disease	CNS tumours
CCNU (1, 2 chloroethyl-, 3 cyclohexyl nitrosourea	oral	Myelosuppression (delayed) Nausea and vomiting Hepatic	Cycle specific	CNS tumours Hodgkin's disease Lymphoma	
Steroids					
Prednisone	oral	Cushing's syndrome Diabetes mellitus Hypertension	Unknown	Acute leukaemia Lymphosarcoma Hodgkin's disease	Histiocytosis X
Epipodophyllins					
VM26	i.v.	Myelosuppression	Unknown	Ewing's sarcoma Soft tissue sarcomas Acute leukaemia	
VP16	i.v.	Myelosuppression	Unknown	Soft tissue sarcomas Acute monocytic leukaemia	

In the majority of tumours where chemotherapy is considered essential, combination chemotherapy should be used combining two, three or more agents, with differing modes of action and differing toxicities in order to obtain the greatest possible anti-tumour effect. In some tumours, e.g. Wilms', where the results of treatment with surgery and combination chemotherapy are highly effective, there are now clinical trials investigating the role of single drug adjuvant chemotherapy.

GENERAL DESCRIPTION OF CHEMOTHERAPEUTIC AGENTS

Many chemotherapeutic agents are now available and a description of all is beyond the scope of this book. A simple classification divides them into:

1 Alkylating agents, e.g. cyclophosphamide, nitrogen mustard.
2 Anti-metabolites, e.g. methotrexate, 5-fluorouracil, mercaptopurine.
3 Antibiotics, e.g. actinomycin-D, daunomycin, adriamycin, bleomycin.
4 Plant alkaloids, e.g. vincristine, vinblastine.
5 Enzymes, e.g. asparaginase.
6 Steroids.
7 Miscellaneous, e.g. hydroxyurea, nitrosoureas, procarbazine.

To use chemotherapy effectively, knowledge of the methods of action, pharmacokinetics, cell kinetics and optimal route and timing of administration of drugs, is essential. It must be borne in mind that not all malignant cells are proliferating at the same rate, and that not all drugs are equally effective throughout the cell cycle. The cell cycle consists of several distinct phases. The relevance of the cell cycle to chemotherapy of leukaemia is described in Chapter 7. To permit continuity of description, some of this information is repeated. Cell division occurs during the mitotic or M phase, which is further subdivided into prophase, metaphase, anaphase and telophase. Following this is a presynthetic gap or G_1 phase, which is a period of active RNA and protein synthesis. This phase controls the duration of the cell cycle. Marked prolongation of this phase is sometimes referred to as the resting or G_0 phase (Fig. 7.1).

In this G_0 phase, cells are not sensitive to cell-cycle specific drugs and therefore form a major barrier to effective chemotherapy. Emerging from G_1, the cells begin a phase of active DNA synthesis termed the S phase. In this period, the DNA complement is duplicated. The cell then enters the post-synthetic or G_2 phase before initiation of mitosis. The length of time for a cell to progress from one mitosis to the next is termed the generation time (Tg). The fraction of cells actively proliferating is termed the growth fraction (Gf).

Chemotherapeutic agents, as well as having differing biochemical mechanisms of action, can be classified according to their effect on cell growth and replication at different phases in the cell cycle. *Cycle specific* agents affect all cells which are in the proliferative cycle, but are without effect on resting (G_0) cells. Examples are cyclophosphamide and 5-fluorouracil. These agents are best administered intermittently at intervals sufficient to allow host recovery in normal tissues. *Phase specific* agents destroy cells only in a particular phase of the cell cycle, most often in the S phase; occasionally G_2, M or G_1. Examples are vincristine, cytosine arabinoside, methotrexate and anthracyclines. For optimal therapy, these agents are given repeatedly so that all proliferating cells are exposed to the drug as they enter the sensitive phase of the cycle.

The concepts outlined above, and in Chapter 7, have been derived from studies with animal models which do not necessarily resemble human malignancy. Much of the information gained from animal studies, however, has been applied successfully to clinical practice. Cancer chemotherapy is still empirical and the optimal route, schedule, duration of treatment and best combination of agents, is yet to be established for the majority of tumours. The reader who desires more detailed information, is referred to the following reviews, while Table 16.2 provides a brief resume of the class, mode of action and tumour sensitivity of the different classes of chemotherapeutic agents.

Side-effects of chemotherapy

Side-effects of chemotherapy are an important consideration in their use. Some of these are common to many agents, e.g. myelosuppression, nausea and vomiting, mucosal ulceration and hair loss. Some are specific to certain agents, e.g. cardiotoxicity secondary to anthracyclines, pulmonary fibrosis secondary to bleomycin and haemorrhagic cystitis secondary to cyclophosphamide. Myelosuppression is the major factor that determines intensity and frequency of treatment. A general rule is that chemotherapy should be suspended if the absolute neutrophil count falls below 1000/μl and/or the platelet count falls below 100 000/μl. The immunosuppressive effects of chemotherapy regimens are also important and opportunistic fungal, protozoal and viral infections are becoming increasingly important complications. Specific details regarding chemotherapy will be found in chapters dealing with individual tumour types.

Equally important as surgery, radiation therapy and chemotherapy, are the psychological, social and economic cost of the disease and its treatment to the child and his/her family. These are dealt with more fully in a later chapter.

RECOMMENDED READING

DeVita V.T., Young R.C. & Canellos G.P. (1975) Combination versus single agent chemotherapy: A review of the basis for selection of drug treatment of cancer. *Cancer* **35**, 98.

Hammond G.D., Bleyer W.A., Hartmann J.R., Hays D.M. & Jenkin R.D.T. (1978) The team approach to the management of paediatric cancer. *Cancer* **41**, 29.

Haseloe R.E., Nesbit M., Dehner L.P., Khan F.M., McHugh F.M. & Levitt S.H. (1978) Second neoplasms following megavoltage radiation in a paediatric population. *Cancer* **42**, 1185.

MEADOWS A.T., D'ANGIO G.J., MIKE V., BANFI A., HARRIS C., JENKIN R.D.T. & SCHWARTZ A., (1977) Patterns of second malignant neoplasms in children. *Cancer* **40**, 1903.
SCHEIN P.S. & WINOKUR S.H. (1975) Immunosuppressive and cytotoxic chemotherapy: Long term complications. *Annals of Internal Medicine* **82**, 84.
SKIPPER H.E. (1978) Adjuvant chemotherapy. *Cancer* **41**, 936.
ZUBROD C.G. (1978) Selective toxicity of anticancer drugs. *Cancer Research* **38**, 4377.

Chapter 17
The Lymphomas

The traditional classification of lymphomas into non-Hodgkin's lymphoma (or lymphosarcoma) and Hodgkin's disease or lymphoma has led to much confusion. The two disorders are not related and should be considered as entirely separate disorders from clinical, investigational, epidemiological and treatment points of view. Similarly, the adult and paediatric forms of each disorder manifest different clinical patterns of behaviour and the paediatric disorder requires an entirely different investigational and treatment programme to that of the adult.

HODGKIN'S DISEASE

Hodgkin's disease is an uncommon disorder in children. It is particularly rare in children less than 5 years of age. Boys are affected 3–4 times more frequently than girls in the younger age groups, but, in older children, there is an approximately equal sex ratio. Three epidemiological types can be recognized. The first is that classically seen in urban western society, with a high rate in young adults and an excess of favourable histological subtypes. The second occurs in developing countries, with high rates in children and a preponderance of unfavourable histological subtypes. The third type occurs in rural western society with an incidence rate intermediate between the first two types. The aetiology of Hodgkin's disease is unknown.

Pathology

Microscopically, four subtypes are recognized.

1 Nodular sclerosing, characterized by the formation of fibrous tissue and Reed-Sternberg cells which lie in lacunae.

2 Lymphocyte predominant type where sheets of abnormal lymphoid cells replace the normal nodal architecture.

3 Mixed cellularity type with marked variation in tissue pattern, cell type and morphology.

4 Lymphocyte depleted with diffuse fibrosis, Reed-Sternberg cells but few lymphocytes.

Adequate surgical sampling of enlarged nodes is essential for accurate histological diagnosis. The biopsy should be an excisional biopsy of a central node which has rapidly enlarged. Biopsy of a satellite node may reveal only reactive hyperplasia.

Presentation

Painless enlarging lymphadenopathy, usually in the cervical region, is the most common presenting symptom. General systemic symptoms (i.e. 'B' symptoms) such as fever, night sweats, anorexia and pruritus, are present in 15–30% of patients, more commonly in Stage III and Stage IV disease. The superior vena cava syndrome may be the mode of onset. Rarely does pressure on, or infiltration of, other organs cause presenting symptoms. Physical findings are those of lymphadenopathy, discrete and shotty in the early stages, but firm and matted at the usual time of presentation. Splenomegaly and/or hepatomegaly may be present, but these findings do not automatically indicate infiltration by Hodgkin's disease (see later).

Investigations

1 Chest X-ray, occasionally proceeding to CAT scan of lungs.
2 FBE and platelet count, ESR.
3 IVP and sometimes bilateral lymphangiography. This procedure may be replaced by a CAT scan or abdominal ultrasound.
4 Urea, creatinine, LFT's, alkaline phosphatase, serum copper.
5 Radioisotope scans (optional) of liver and spleen and nodes.
6 Staging laparotomy with splenectomy and bone marrow biopsy (? optional).

Staging

Accurate staging of the extent of disease was advocated when it was realized that Hodgkin's disease tends to spread in a predictable fashion to adjacent

Table 17.1 Staging of Hodgkin's disease (Ann Arbor system).

Stage I
Involvement of a single lymph node region (I) or a single extralymphatic site (Ie).

Stage II
Involvement of two or more node areas on the same side of the diaphragm (II) or localized involvement of an extralymphatic site and one or more lymph node regions on the same side of the diaphragm (IIe).

Stage III
Involvement of lymph nodes on both sides of the diaphragm (III) which may be accompanied by involvement of the spleen (IIIs) or by localized involvement of an extralymphatic organ or site (IIIe) or both (IIIse).

Stage IV
Diffuse or disseminated involvement of one or more extralymphatic organs or tissues with or without associated lymph node involvement.

nodes, and that with 'therapeutic' irradiation to the involved area only, relapse often occurred in the immediately adjacent nodal areas.

Similarly, the high rate of occult abdominal nodal and splenic involvement makes accurate assessment of the extent of the disease essential if irradiation therapy alone is the mode of treatment. Initial work-up involves assignment of a clinical stage (CS). Following staging laparotomy and splenectomy, a pathological stage (PS) can be assigned. The Ann Arbor staging system is commonly used and is shown in Table 17.1.

Staging laparotomy in children should not be considered a routine procedure. It is of no value when there is definite evidence of Stage III or IV Hodgkin's disease, e.g. obvious involvement of lymph node areas above and below the diaphragm with or without hepatosplenomegaly, or in patients with lung or bone marrow infiltration. There can be little debate about its value in other children, as there is a 30% incidence of incorrect clinical staging, but only if the stage of the disease influences the treatment. If a uniform treatment programme is adopted for all children irrespective of stage, then a staging laparotomy is not necessary. There is no doubt that staging laparotomy with splenectomy is associated with a significant morbidity and mortality as a result of overwhelming bacterial infections.

Treatment

IRRADIATION THERAPY

The dramatic improvement in results of treatment of Hodgkin's disease initially resulted from the application of radical radiation therapy techniques ranging from upper mantle or inverted Y fields to total nodal irradiation. These techniques can be applied to children, but there are undesirable immediate and long-term side-effects which are: immunosuppression; growth failure; soft tissue and muscle atrophy; and the carcinogenic potential of irradiation. The current trend in childhood Hodgkin's disease is therefore to rely on chemotherapy as the mainstay of treatment and to use radiotherapy on a 'supplementary' basis only.

Adequate curative doses of irradiation for childhood Hodgkin's disease are 35–40 Gy given over 3–4 weeks, with appropriate shielding of vital structures such as the larynx, lungs, liver and kidneys. With the advent of more effective chemotherapy, it may be possible to modify doses and reduce field sizes to involved areas only, and early results do not indicate that survival is jeopardized.

CHEMOTHERAPY

Many single agents are effective in Hodgkin's disease, with responses varying from 10 to 80%. These responses are invariably of short duration. The introduction of the highly successful combination of nitrogen mustard, vincristine, prednisolone and procarbazine (MOPP) led to the widespread use of combination chemotherapy combining active antitumour agents with differing toxicities. The standard against which all other chemotherapy programmes must be assessed remains MOPP. With MOPP, an 80% remission rate, with an actuarial median survival in excess of 5 years, has been achieved. Other combination programmes are best reserved for MOPP failures or for patients who relapse following initial successful primary therapy. These are shown in Table 17.2. Although the question of 'maintenance therapy' is still unresolved, it is our practice to give an additional six courses of maintenance MOPP at 6 weekly intervals for Stage III and Stage IV disease.

In view of the efficacy of MOPP alone in Stage IV disease, it would seem appropriate to explore the use of chemotherapy alone in the treatment for State I and Stage II disease.

As with irradiation, chemotherapy also has undesirable side-effects and should only be undertaken in experienced units. Apart from myelotoxicity and immunosuppression, there is evidence that, in adults, MOPP chemotherapy results in total or partial sterility. The effect of MOPP

Table 17.2 Combination chemotherapy in Hodgkin's disease.

MOPP
Nitrogen mustard 6 mg/m^2 i.v. days 1 and 8
Vincristine 1.5 mg/m^2 i.v. days 1 and 8
Procarbazine 100 mg/m^2/day orally days 1–15
Prednisolone 50 mg/m^2/day orally days 1–15
Repeated every 28 days as tolerated

MVPP
As above, except vinblastine 6 mg/m^2 i.v. on days 1 and 8 is substituted for vincristine

ABVD
Adriamycin 25 mg/m^2 i.v. days 1 and 14
Bleomycin 10 mg/m^2 i.v. days 1 and 14
Vinblastine 6 mg/m^2 i.v. days 1 and 14
DIC 150 mg/m^2 i.v. days 1–5
Repeated every 28 days as tolerated

CAVE
CCNU 100 mg/m^2 orally day 1
Adriamycin 60 mg/m^2 i.v. day 1
Vinblastine 5 mg/m^2 i.v. day 1
Repeated every 6 weeks as tolerated

Cyclophosphamide 600 mg/m^2 i.v. on days 1 and 8 can be substituted for nitrogen mustard in the MOPP and MVPP regimens.
Chlorambucil 6 mg/m^2/day orally days 1–15 can be substituted for nitrogen mustard in the MOPP and MVPP regimens.

chemotherapy on fertility, when given to prepubertal children, has not been adequately investigated, but there must be a suspicion that fertility will be reduced.

Prognosis

Survival figures for children are at least as good as those for adult patients. For Stage I and Stage II patients, a 5 year survival of 90% is expected with current treatment. For Stage III patients, 70–80% 5 year survival, and for Stage IV patients, at least 50% 5 year survival, is expected. In most recent series, early mortality has occurred mainly from toxic effects of chemotherapy rather than relapse of the disease.

NON-HODGKIN'S LYMPHOMA (LYMPHOSARCOMA)

Occurs at all ages in childhood, although very rarely below the age of 3 years. Boys are affected two to three times more commonly than girls. Lymphosarcoma in childhood bears little relationship to lymphosarcoma in adults for the following reasons:

1 High frequency of marrow and/or CNS involvement during the course of the disease (e.g. up to 80% in patients with mediastinal presentation).

2 Extreme rarity of nodular and mixed lymphocytic/histiocytic histologic subtypes in children (nearly all cases are of diffuse, poorly differentiated histology).

3 Blurring of the distinction between lymphosarcoma with marrow involvement and true acute lymphocytic leukaemia of childhood.

Pathology

The most widely used system of classification is that devised by Rappaport which categorizes lymphomas on the basis of pattern, nodular or diffuse, and cytology, lymphocytic, histiocytic or mixed. This classification has been modified for paediatric tumours and has proven useful with respect to treatment and prognosis. The modification of the Rappaport classification used by the Children's Cancer Study Group is outlined below.

1 Poorly differentiated diffuse lymphoblastic lymphoma.

2 Burkitt's tumour.

3 Undifferentiated non-Burkitt's.

4 Large cell or histiocytic lymphoma.

The Rappaport classification was devised before development of knowledge and techniques of measuring the derivation of lymphoid cells from T- and B-cell lines (Chapter 7). It has also been firmly established that the histiocytic lymphomas are predominantly neoplasms of large transformed lymphocytes and that true tumours of histiocytes are very rare.

Alternative classifications have been proposed by other workers, of which the Lukes-Collins system has gained the widest acceptance. This classification is based on morphologic and immunologic features, but at the present time, correlation of the classification with clinical studies is restricted to relatively small numbers of patients. New technology, particularly the use of monoclonal antibodies for lymphocyte subtypes, will almost certainly alter the classification of lymphomas once again.

At the present time, the Rappaport classification remains the most widely used and, to some extent, it can be correlated with cell marker characteristics. Thus, the poorly differentiated lymphoblastic lymphomas are most often of the T-cell type, particularly if the cells show morphologic features of convoluted nuclei. Some of these lymphomas are neither T nor B and may have cell surface marker characteristics similar to childhood cALL. Burkitt's lymphomas show B-cell marker characteristics. The undifferentiated non-Burkitt's lymphomas are a heterogenous group not well correlated with surface cell markers. The large cell or histiocytic lymphomas are usually of the B-cell type.

Clinical staging is of confirmed value and the system proposed by Murphy is shown in Table 17.3. In patients with mediastinal lymphoma, every effort should be made to obtain histiological confirmation of the diagnosis, even to the extent of performing a thoracotomy, before commencing treatment.

Spread

Infiltration of the marrow may be already present at diagnosis. Patients with over 25–40% marrow infiltration are often considered to have acute leukaemia. Marrow spread occurs in up to 40% of patients during the evolution of their disease. CNS involvement occurs in 30% of lymphosarcoma overall, but ranging from less than 10% in patients with primary abdominal disease to 80–90% in patients with T-cell lymphoma and mediastinal or cervical primaries. Testicular infiltration is also relatively common in the T-cell group.

Clinical features

The clinical picture varies according to the primary site and extent of disease. Regional or generalized enlargement of peripheral lymph nodes may be obvious. Mediastinal involvement may present with acute superior vena caval obstruction or signs and symptoms of a pleural effusion. Abdominal pain and signs of an intussusception or partial or complete bowel obstruction indicate the presence of abdominal involvement. These lesions characteristically present as one of two extremes, viz. as a localized readily removable lesion usually causing intussusception or as massive intra-abdominal disease with peritoneal fluid, the site of origin being indeterminate. Abdominal disease is the commonest primary site accounting for 30–40% of cases.

In Caucasians, widespread abdominal or ovarian lymphoma is frequently of the Burkitt type. The type of lymphosarcoma involving the jaw and presenting as large facial destructive masses, described by Burkitt, is very infrequent outside Africa and New Guinea. The differential diagnosis of lymphoma from leukaemia is particularly difficult. There is a tendency to define lymphoma as mass disease with haemoglobin greater than 10 g% and no circulating leukaemic cells, irrespective of the degree of bone marrow infiltration.

Staging

The extent of disease at diagnosis naturally determines the treatment required and the patient's prognosis. The Ann Arbor staging system is not particularly appropriate to childhood lymphosarcoma, as discussed in the introduction, and for this reason, the St Jude staging system shown in Table 17.3 is more appropriate.

Investigations required are full blood and platelet count, chest X-ray and skeletal survey, multiple bone marrow aspiration and trephine, to rule out patchy marrow infiltration, and CSF examination. Rarely, bipedal lymph-angiography and IVP may be performed. CAT scans are frequently useful to assess the extent of disease. Staging laparotomy and splenectomy are of no use in determining treatment.

Table 17.3 Staging of childhood lymphosarcoma (Murphy system)

Stage I
A single tumour (extra nodal) or single anatomic area (nodal) excluding mediastinum or abdomen

Stage II
A single tumour (extra nodal) with regional node involvement.
Two or more nodal areas on the same side of the diaphragm. A resectable primary gastrointestinal tumour with or without associated mesenteric node involvement

Stage III
Two single tumours on opposite sides of the diaphragm.
Two or more nodal areas above and below the diaphragm.
All the primary intrathoracic tumours.
All extensive unresectable abdominal disease

Stage IV
Any of the above with initial involvement of the bone marrow and/or central nervous system

Treatment

The intensity of the treatment varies with the site and stage of the tumour. All patients should be approached with curative intent at diagnosis.

SURGERY

Apart from removal of localized abdominal lesions, the role of surgery is limited to biopsy of involved nodes. In patients with gross irremovable abdominal disease initially, early second-look surgery with removal of residual disease has been advocated by some as an effective means of therapy.

IRRADIATION THERAPY

Because lymphosarcoma is never truly 'localized', irradiation alone is inadequate as a form of curative treatment. Lymphosarcoma is a radiosensitive lesion and local node masses will quickly respond to 30–35 Gy given over 3–4 weeks. There is no benefit to be gained from therapeutic irradiation of mediastinal lesions because it causes profound immunosuppression and because, most often, systemic rather than local relapses occur in those patients who fail therapy. Emergency low dose irradiation, e.g. 3–4 Gy, may be necessary to relieve obstructive symptoms, although it is general experience that chemotherapy is equally and as rapidly effective.

Patients with completely resectable abdominal primaries do not require irradiation therapy to the abdomen or CNS prophylaxis. In patients with positive mesenteric node involvement or with residual gross disease, total abdominal irradiation to a dose of 25–30 Gy may be given with appropriate shielding of liver and kidneys. Local coned irradiation to grossly involved areas may be continued to a dose of 35–40 Gy.

For patients requiring CNS prophylaxis (viz. all except patients with abdominal disease), 18 or 24 Gy of craniocervical irradiation is given as for patients with ALL (see chapter 7). In some centres, CNS prophylaxis is not given for patients with Stage I disease.

CHEMOTHERAPY

Chemotherapy is the mainstay of treatment in childhood lymphosarcoma. Many agents have activity, most useful being: vincristine, prednisolone, high dose cyclophosphamide, anthracyclines and moderate or high dose methotrexate. Most programmes combine these agents in an intermittent fashion. Single agent therapy is ineffective.

As for acute lymphocytic leukaemia, the first objective is to obtain a complete remission. Remission rates of 85–90% can be achieved with most lymphomas, except in those patients with widespread abdominal disease with or without marrow infiltration where the remission rates are approximately 50%. Following induction of remission, some form of continuation therapy

Table 17.4 Combination chemotherapy in non-Hodgkin's lymphoma.

CHOP
Vincristine 1.5 mg/m^2 i.v.
Cyclophosphamide 600–1200 mg/m^2 i.v.
Adriamycin 60 mg/m^2 i.v.
Prednisolone 50 mg/m^2 orally for 5 days

COMP
Vincristine 1.5 mg/m^2 i.v.
Cyclophosphamide 1.0–1.2 g/m^2 i.v.
Methotrexate 300 mg/m^2 (60% of dose as injection, 40% as a 4 hour infusion)
Prednisolone 60 mg/m^2 orally for 5 days

Table 17.5 LSA_2–L_2 protocol (modified to reduce toxicity).

Induction
Cyclophosphamide 1.2 g/m^2 i.v.
Vincristine 2 mg/m^2 i.v.
Daunomycin 60 mg/m^2 i.v.
Prednisolone 60 mg/m^2 orally for 4 weeks
Intrathecal methotrexate 6.25 mg/m^2

Consolidation
Ara-C 100 mg/m^2 daily for 5 days
6-thioguanine 50 mg/m^2 8–12 hourly after Ara-C injection
L-asparaginase 6000 μ/m^2/d for 14 days after completion of Ara-C and 6-thioguanine
Intrathecal methotrexate 6.25 mg/m^2 twice, 3 days apart, after completion of L-asparaginase
BCNU 60 mg/m^2 i.v. 2–3 days after completion of methotrexate

Maintenance
5 day cycles followed by rest period to recovery of blood count:

1 6-thioguanine 300 mg/m^2 orally for 4 days followed by cyclophosphamide 600 mg/m^2 on day 5

2 Hydroxyurea 2.4 g/m^2 orally for 4 days followed by daunomycin 45 mg/m^2 on day 5

3 Methotrexate 10 mg/m^2 daily for 4 days followed by BCNU 60 mg/m^2 i.v. on day 5

4 Ara-C 150 mg/m^2 i.v. daily for 4 days followed by vincristine 2 mg/m^2 (maximum dose 2 mg) on day 5

5 Intrathecal methotrexate 6.25 mg/m^2 two doses 3 days apart must be given. This may vary from a simple two drug maintenance regimen (6-MP and methotrexate) for Stage I and II disease, to intensive cycles of multiple drugs similar to those used for induction. In some centres, no continuation therapy is given for patients with Burkitt's tumour following the initial 6 month 'induction' period. In this group of patients, CNS prophylaxis has not been fully effective in preventing CNS relapse. Various protocols of treatment utilizing multiple agent chemotherapy can be obtained from major oncological centres. The best known are those characterized by the acronyms, CHOP, COMP and LSA_2-L_2. They should only be used by experienced oncologists and the details of their administration must be obtained from relevant protocols designed by these institutions. The drugs used in CHOP and COMP are shown in Table 17.4. The LSA_2-L_2 protocol is summarized in Table 17.5 and is described in the reference of Wollner *et al.* (1975).

Prognosis

Prior to the introduction of an aggressive multimodal approach as outlined above, survival for childhood lymphosarcoma was approximately 30%. With current therapy, 2 year disease-free survivals of 80% are expected for Stage I and Stage II patients, and of 30–50% for Stage III and Stage IV patients. It is very uncommon for recurrence to occur after a 2 year disease-free period. There is evidence that the undifferentiated lymphoblastic lymphomas respond best to the LSA_2-L_2 type protocols, while the other types of non-Hodgkin's lymphoma respond better to COMP type regimens.

The prognosis of all the lymphomas (except Burkitt's), which present with mass lesions above the diaphragm or with diffuse nodular disease without abdominal involvement, is better than those of Burkitt's tumour or undifferentiated non-Burkitt's, which present with widespread abdominal disease.

RECOMMENDED READING

Hodgkin's disease

Botnick L.E., Goodman R., Jaffe N., Filler R. & Cassady J.R. (1977) Stages I–III Hodgkin's disease in children. Results of staging and treatment. *Cancer* **39**, 599.

Cadman E.C., Capizzi R.L. & Bertino J.R. (1977) Acute nonlymphatic leukaemia. A delayed complication of Hodgkin's disease therapy: analysis of 109 cases. *Cancer* **40**, 1280.

Desforges J.F. & Rutherford C.J. (1979) Hodgkin's disease. *New England Journal of Medicine* **301**, 1212.

Donaldson S.S., Glatstein E. & Vosti K.L. (1978) Bacterial infections in paediatric Hodgkin's disease. Relationship to radiotherapy, chemotherapy and splenectomy. *Cancer* **41**, 1949.

JENKIN D., FREEDMAN M., MCCLURE P., PETERS V., SAUNDERS F. & SONLEY M. (1979) Hodgkin's disease in children: Treatments with low dose radiation and MOPP without staging laparotomy. A preliminary report. *Cancer* **44**, 80.

LANGE S., LITTMAN P., SCHNAUFER L. & EVANS A.E. (1978) Treatment of advanced Hodgkin's disease in paediatric patients. *Cancer* **42**, 1141.

OLWENY C.L.M., KATONGOLE-MBIDDE E., KIIRE C., LWANGA S.K., MAGRATH I. & ZIEGLER J.L. (1978) Childhood Hodgkin's disease in Uganda. A ten year experience. *Cancer* **42**, 787.

Non-Hodgkin's lymphoma

APPELBAUM F.R., HERZIG G.P., ZIEGLER J.L., GRAW R.G., LEVINE A.S. & DEISSEROTH A.B. (1978) Successful engraftment of cryopreserved autologous bone marrow in patients with malignant lymphoma. *Blood* **52**, 85.

BRECHER M.L., SINKS L.F., THOMAS R.R.M. & FREEMAN A.I. (1978) Non-Hodgkin's lymphoma in children. *Cancer* **41**, 1997.

CARABELL S.G., CASSADY J.R., WEINSTEIN H. & JAFFE N. (1978) The role of radiation therapy in the treatment of paediatric non-Hodgkin's lymphoma. *Cancer* **42**, 2193.

MURPHY S.B. (1978) Childhood non-Hodgkin's lymphoma. *New England Journal of Medicine* **299**, 1446.

WEINSTEIN H.J., VANCE Z.B., JAFFE N., BUELL D., CASSADY J.R. & NATHAN D.G. (1979) Improved prognosis for patients with mediastinal lymphoblastic lymphoma. *Blood* **53**, 687.

WILLIAMS A.H., TAYLOR C.A., HIGGINS G.R., QUINN J.J., SCHNEIDER B.K., SWANSON V., PARKER J.W., PATTENGALE P.K., CHANDOR S.B., POWARS D., LINCOLN T.L., TINDLE B.H. & LUKES R.J. (1978) Childhood lymphoma — leukaemia. 1. Correlation of morphology and immunologic studies. *Cancer* **42**, 171.

WOLLNER N., BURCHENAL J.H., LIEBERMAN P.H., EXELBY P.R., D'ANGIO G.J. & MURPHY M.L. (1975) Non-Hodgkin's lymphoma in children. *Medical and Pediatric Oncology* **1**, 235.

ZIEGLER J.L. (1977) Treatment results of 54 American patients with Burkitt's lymphoma are similar to the African experience. *New England Journal of Medicine* **297**, 75.

Chapter 18
Wilms' Tumour

Wilms' tumour accounts for 5–10% of paediatric solid malignancies. It is the cornerstone on which the foundation of paediatric oncology has been built. With surgical removal of the primary alone, survival rates of 20% were achieved. Following the introduction of postoperative irradiation therapy, a survival rate of 40% was obtained. Repeated courses of adjuvant chemotherapy with vincristine and actinomycin D have now improved the 2 year survival rate to 80–90%.

General characteristics

Wilms' tumour occurs most commonly in the first 5 years of life, with a slight predominance in males over females. The left kidney is involved slightly more frequently than the right. The incidence of bilateral tumours varies markedly, from 3–12% in reported series. Whether this represents simultaneous multiple primaries or metastatic spread from one kidney to another, remains an unanswered question.

Certain congenital abnormalities are associated with an increased frequency of Wilms' tumour. These are, hemihypertrophy, aniridia, Beckwith syndrome and genitourinary anomalies.

Pathological characteristics

Most consist of a single mass, central or polar in location, surrounded by a pseudocapsule of fibrous tissue and compressed renal parenchyma. The cut surface is greyish-pink with myxomatous haemorrhagic and necrotic areas. Local extension through the renal capsule may involve perinephric fat, retroperitoneal tissues, adrenal gland, diaphragm, liver and bowel. Involvement of hilar and periaortic nodes occurs in some 15% of patients and appears to be associated with a decreased survival rate.

Histological examination reveals a biphasic pattern of epithelial and mesenchymal elements. There is substantial evidence that certain histological features are associated with a favourable response to treatment, while others are associated with poor response to currently practised therapeutic regimens. Most pathologists agree that evidence of tubular or glomerular differentiation are favourable histological signs. Some consider that any form of differentiation, including that into muscle fibres or adipose tissue, are also favourable. It is generally agreed that a lack of differentiation with the presence in blastema or cells with giant nuclei is an unfavourable histological feature.

It is essential to separate the entity of mesoblastic nephroma (or fetal renal hamartoma) from Wilms' tumour. These tumours may be very large, but seldom metastasize. Cure may be achieved with surgical removal alone, but as local recurrence has been described, adjuvant chemotherapy may be indicated. They are commonly found within the first few months of life.

The commonest site of metastases is the lungs. Haematogenous spread to the liver is less common, while metastases to the skeleton and central nervous system are uncommon, except in terminal cases.

Presenting features

The patients most commonly present because of accidental discovery of an asymptomatic abdominal mass. Less frequently, abdominal pain may lead to the discovery of an abdominal mass. Haematuria is an uncommon occurrence. Hypertension may be associated with the tumour, but is rarely a presenting feature. Very infrequently, there may be sudden or traumatic tumour rupture leading to abdominal pain and shock. The differential diagnosis includes polycystic kidneys, hydronephrosis, neuroblastoma, hepatoblastoma and adrenal carcinoma. In left-sided Wilms' tumour, it is sometimes difficult to differentiate between a renal tumour and splenomegaly. In such cases, radiologic investigations settle the issue.

Investigations

These are designed to define the site and extent of the local tumour and whether spread to distant sites has occurred. The basic investigations are plain X-rays of abdomen, chest and intravenous pyelogram. The local extent of the tumour can be defined by an abdominal CAT scan or ultrasound, which may also demonstrate enlarged lymph nodes. If there are suspicious lung lesions on plain chest X-ray, they may be better defined by CAT scan of the chest. As a routine, skeletal survey or bone scans are not necessary. However, in tumours with unfavourable histology, one or other should be performed.

Aortography, selective renal angiography and inferior venocavography are only indicated in the rare instances where the surgeon requires a precise knowledge of the blood supply of the tumour for its removal. Cavography may be particularly useful in patients in whom there is a suspicion that tumour growth has extended from the renal vein into the inferior vena cava. Ultrasound has replaced these invasive investigations.

Staging

Various staging systems have been proposed. The National Wilms' Tumour

Study Group (NWTS) in the USA, which uses clinical groups rather than stages, is probably the most appropriate, Accurate 'grouping' requires the close cooperation of the clinician, surgeon and pathologist, as the degree and intensity of chemotherapy and radiotherapy will be determined by the final group allocation. The NWTS staging system is shown in Table 18.1.

Treatment

Each of the three disciplines of surgery, radiotherapy and chemotherapy play an important role. Each will be considered separately. Preliminary clinical assessment will allow a tentative clinical group to be assigned. Final classification, and therefore definitive treatment, depends upon both the surgical and pathological findings.

SURGERY

Total removal of the involved kidney should be the aim for all patients with Wilms' tumour. For experienced paediatric surgeons, a Wilms' tumour is rarely inoperable. A transabdominal or abdominothoracic approach is used with early ligation of the renal vessels. The primary tumour is removed intact. The contralateral kidney, the liver and abdominal cavity should be carefully inspected for evidence of tumour. There is no general agreement on lymph node sampling. All surgeons agree that suspicious nodes in the renal hilum or periaortic regions should be excised. In the absence of suspicious nodes, it may be reasonable to biopsy accessible lymph nodes, but a total node clearance should not be attempted. The value of random lymph node sampling as an aid to accurate staging is not established.

Table 18.1 Staging of Wilms' tumour.

Group I
Tumour limited to kidney and completely resected

Group II
Tumour extends beyond kidney (penetration beyond pseudocapsule, periaortic node involvement, renal vessel involvement beyond kidney), but is completely resected

Group III
Residual non-haematogenous tumour confined to abdomen, e.g. tumour rupture before or during surgery, tumour not completely resectable, nodes beyond periaortic chain involved

Group IV
Haematogenous metastases

Group V
Bilateral renal involvement, either initially or subsequently

In some centres, preoperative irradiation or chemotherapy is given to shrink the tumour and make it more easily operable. The results of the International Society of Paediatric Oncology (SIOP) trial showed no difference in survival or recurrence-free survival in patients randomized to receive or not receive preoperative irradiation therapy. One risk of such an approach is that patients with benign disorders may be given unnecessary therapy.

IRRADIATION

Historically, improvements in prognosis of Wilms' tumour followed the introduction of postoperative irradiation to the tumour bed. Initially, all patients were treated. Results of the NWTS have now shown that postoperative irradiation therapy to the tumour bed is unnecessary for patients with favourable histology and Group I tumours. With multiple drug chemotherapy, it may also prove to be unnecessary in Group II tumours. On the other hand, postoperative irradiation is required for all patients with unfavourable histology irrespective of clinical grouping. Group III patients are treated with postoperative irradiation therapy, which usually commences immediately histological confirmation of the diagnosis is obtained. The renal bed, and the entire width of the vertebral bodies, is treated. The dose given varies according to the age of the child, as shown in Table 18.2.

In Group III patients with gross peritoneal contamination, total abdominal irradiation is necessary. Tumour rupture during operation with spill into the tumour bed is not an indication for total abdominal irradiation. The field should extend from the diaphragm to the obturator foramen, with shielding of the femoral heads. In Group IV patients with pulmonary metastases, the usual practice is to give bilateral lung field irradiation to a dose not exceeding 20 Gy. There may be a role for avoiding lung field irradiation, provided complete control can be achieved with intensive chemotherapy and/or surgical resection.

CHEMOTHERAPY

The mainstays of treatment are a combination of vincristine and actinomycin D. More recently, adriamycin has also been demonstrated to be an effective agent in the treatment of Wilms' tumour. Historically, actinomycin D was the first drug with demonstrable anti-Wilms' tumour activity. Subsequently,

Table 18.2 Irradiation therapy dose regimens for Wilms' tumour.

Age (months)	Dose
0–18	18–24 Gy
19–30	24–30 Gy
31–40	30–35 Gy
41+	35–40 Gy

vincristine was also shown to be effective, and a combination of both drugs was more effective than either used as a single agent. These studies were performed before it was realized that the histological features of the tumour were associated with prognosis. Large national studies in the USA, UK and Europe are now reassessing the need for intensive and multiple drug maintenance and the optimal duration of treatment.

For Group I tumours with favourable histology, there is now evidence that 6 months of chemotherapy with vincristine and actinomycin D constitutes adequate therapy, with 90% disease-free survival rates. Further investigations are underway to limit combination chemotherapy to only two courses of actinomycin D and 10 weekly injections of vincristine. The use of single agent chemotherapy is also under investigation and early results appear promising.

For tumours with favourable histology and in Group II or III, the usual duration of therapy is 15 months, with intermittent courses of actinomycin D and vincristine usually given at 9–13 week intervals. The role of additional adriamycin is under investigation.

For tumours with unfavourable histology or favourable histology but Group IV, the usual duration of chemotherapy is 15 months, with intermittent courses of vincristine, actinomycin D and adriamycin. The value of this drug regimen in patients with unfavourable histology is unproven. The usual doses of drugs are:

Vincristine 1.5 mg/m^2 (dose not to exceed 2 mg)
Actinomycin D 15 μg/kg/day for 5 days
Adriamycin 20 mg/m^2/day for 3 days.

TOXICITY

Myelosuppression, mouth ulcers, nausea and vomiting and alopecia can be troublesome. Liver function abnormalities occur if the liver is in the field of irradiation. Liver enlargement, jaundice and elevated levels of transaminases are present. Isotope scans show focal cold areas in the liver which can be mistaken for metastatic involvement. Cardiotoxicity is a potential complication of adriamycin usually related to the total dose given. With concurrent mediastinal irradiation, it is not safe to exceed a total dose of 300 mg/m^2 of adriamycin.

BILATERAL WILMS' TUMOUR

No specific regimen can be recommended. Each case must be treated on its merits. Surgical excision should be performed wherever possible. Irradiation is also given, but radiation nephritis of remaining renal tissue must be avoided. Combination chemotherapy with vincristine, actinomycin D and adriamycin may be considered, but is not of established value.

Prognosis

In patients with favourable histology, the disease-free rates at 2 years, using the treatment regimens outlined previously, are as follows:

Group I 95%
Group II 80–90%
Group III 70–85%
Group IV 50–60%

In patients with unfavourable histology, the disease-free rates at 2 years are between 30–50%.

RECOMMENDED READING

BRESLOW N.E., PALMER N.F., HILL L.R., BURING J. & D'ANGIO G.J. (1978) Wilms' tumour: prognostic factors for patients without metastases at diagnosis. Results of the National Wilms' Tumour Study. *Cancer* **41**, 1577.

BECKWITH J.B. & PALMER N.F. (1978) Histopathology and prognosis of Wilms' tumour. Results from the First National Wilms' Tumour Study. *Cancer* **41**, 1937.

CHADAREVIAN J.P., FLETCHER B.D., CHAFFEN J. & ROBINOVITCH H.H. (1977) Massive infantile nephroblastomatosis. *Cancer* **39**, 2294.

D'ANGIO G.J., EVANS A.E., BRESLOW N., BECKWITH B., BISHOP H., FEIGL P., GOODWIN W., LEAPE L.I., SINKS L.F., SUTOW W.W., TEFFT M. & WOLFF J. (1976) The treatment of Wilms' tumour: Results of the National Wilms' Study. *Cancer* **38**, 663.

D'ANGIO G.J., TEFFT M., BRESLOW N. & MEYER J.A. (1978) Radiation therapy of Wilms' tumour: Results according to dose, field, post-operative timing and histology. *International Journal of Radiation, Oncology, Biology, Physics* **4**, 769.

D'ANGIO G.J., BECKWITH J.B., BRESLOW N.E. *et al.* (1980) Wilms' tumour: An update. *Cancer* **45**, 1971.

GREEN D.M. & JAFFE N. (1979) The role of chemotherapy in the treatment of Wilms' Tumour. *Cancer* **44**, 52.

JEREB B., TOURNADE M.F., LEMERLE J. *et al.* (1980) Lymph node invasion and prognosis in nephroblastoma. *Cancer* **45**, 1632.

LEMERLE J., TOURNADE M.F., GERARD-MARCHANT R. *et al.* (1976) Wilms' tumour: natural history and prognostic factors. *Cancer* **37**, 2257.

MARSDEN H.B., LAWLER W. & KUMAR P.M. (1978) Bone metastasizing renal tumour of childhood: morphological and clinical features, and differences from Wilms' tumour. *British Journal of Cancer* **38**, 437.

PRENDERGRASS T.W. (1976) Congenital anomalies in children with Wilms' tumour. A new survey. *Cancer* **37**, 403.

Chapter 19
Neuroblastoma

Neuroblastoma constitutes 7–10% of paediatric solid tumours. The annual incidence is 10/million children under the age of 15 years. It arises from neural crest tissue and can occur at any site along the craniospinal axis. In the majority of patients, it is an extremely aggressive malignancy which is little affected by intensive therapy. However, in infants under the age of 12 months with widespread involvement of skin, liver and bone marrow, there is a spontaneous regression rate of 60%. The factors that lead to spontaneous regression of this tumour are obviously of major importance in understanding its nature and possibly in designing more effective modes of treatment. Unfortunately, despite much research effort, little progress has been made.

Incidence and aetiology

Neuroblastoma occurs predominantly in infancy and childhood; males are affected slightly more frequently than females. The clinical incidence probably represents only the tip of the iceberg, as neuroblastoma *in situ* has been demonstrated in autopsy series with a frequency ranging from 1:50 to 1:250. It is assumed that the majority of these *in situ* tumours undergo spontaneous regression by as yet unknown mechanisms.

Pathologic characteristics

SITES OF ORIGIN

Abdominal tumours account for 50%, the majority being adrenal in origin. Thoracic lesions are paravertebral in situation and may be massive in size before producing symptoms. If 'dumbbell' extension through the intervertebral foramina occurs, neurological disturbances, ranging from bladder and/or bowel dysfunction to complete paraplegia, may be the first manifestation. These tumours are usually nonmetastatic. Pelvic, cervical and head neck primaries are relatively uncommon. In approximately 10%, the primary site of origin is never found.

MACROSCOPIC APPEARANCES

Local tumours are usually well encapsulated and the cut surface is reddish and friable with areas of necrosis and calcification. Retroperitoneal tumours are characteristically locally invasive, being irremovably fixed to the posterior abdominal wall.

HISTOLOGIC APPEARANCES

Malignant neuroblastoma is composed of densely packed small round cells. Neurofibrils and the characteristic rosette appearance occur in the more differentiated tumours, and are most prominent in ganglioneuroblastomas where mature ganglion cells are seen. Ganglioneuroma is a benign tumour which may represent a malignant neuroblastoma which has converted to a benign tumour by unknown mechanisms.

Attempts have been made to grade neuroblastoma on the basis of the degree of differentiation and to relate this to prognosis. Some authors have reported that the more differentiated tumours have a better prognosis. The largest proportion, however, is made up of undifferentiated tumours and the varying proportions of maturing elements could not be related to prognosis.

Presenting features

In approximately 70% of patients, the disease is metastatic at presentation. The symptoms are similar to those in acute leukaemia, with pallor, weight loss, bone pain and recurrent fever being most prominent. Bruising or other haemorrhagic manifestations are rare. Less common but characteristic modes of presentation include unilateral proptosis with upper eyelid bruising, sudden onset of partial or total spinal cord compression and the finding of a posterior mediastinal mass on chest X-ray. In infants under the age of 6 months, the disease may present in a very characteristic manner leading to the term 'blueberry muffin' baby. In these infants, there are multiple subcutaneous nodules of tumour, some of which have a purple hue.

Despite the fact that many neuroblastomas are hormone secreting tumours, symptoms or findings of hypertension or chronic diarrhoea are very rare. Nevertheless, the possibility of neuroblastoma should be considered when hypertension or chronic diarrhoea have no other obvious cause. Another rare manifestation of neuroblastoma is acute cerebellar encephalopathy, accompanied by truncal ataxia and oculogyric crises. This situation is usually associated with an occult neuroblastoma.

Physical examination reveals the primary tumour in 50% of patients. There is often a hard, irregular fixed mass in either the right or left hypochondrium. It is often difficult to distinguish the mass from the kidney, but in the context of the patient's presentation with general malaise, the diagnosis of neuroblastoma is more likely than Wilms' tumour. Lymph node enlargement may also be a prominent feature of neuroblastoma. Cervical and axillary lymph nodes are most often involved, but they are seldom as large as those seen with Hodgkin's or non-Hodgkin's lymphomas. It is apparent from the above description that neuroblastoma more than any other paediatric tumour has protean manifestations. It follows that neuroblastoma should be considered in a very wide variety of presenting symptoms. The most important are:

1 Unexplained anaemia.
2 Fever of unknown origin.
3 Failure to thrive.
4 Limp, generalized bone pain and refusal to walk.
5 Abdominal, pelvic or mediastinal mass.
6 Sudden onset of paraplegia.
7 Proptosis.

Investigations

FULL BLOOD COUNT, PLATELET COUNT AND ESR

Anaemia and thrombocytopenia are manifestations of disseminated disease. The ESR may be a simple, but non-specific, way of monitoring progress.

BONE MARROW EXAMINATION

All patients with proven and suspected neuroblastoma require bone marrow examination for diagnostic and staging purposes. Malignant cells may be dispersed or present in clumps forming 'pseudorosettes'. Occasionally, neurofibrillae are apparent. The presence of both malignant cells in the marrow and elevated urinary catecholamines (see later) constitutes sufficient evidence to establish the diagnosis of neuroblastoma.

RADIOLOGIC INVESTIGATIONS

Calcification on plain films is seen more often in neuroblastoma than other paediatric tumours. The intensity of radiologic investigations depends on the site of the tumour. In abdominal tumours, intravenous pyelogram and CAT scans usually demonstrate the site and size of tumour and have largely replaced the invasive procedures of angiography. With spinal cord compression, myelography as well as CAT scans may be required to define the exact extension of tumour in the spinal canal. In the case of pelvic and mediastinal tumours, CAT scans can define the extent of tumour and, in particular, whether there are dumbbell extensions into the spinal canal. All patients with neuroblastoma should have a skeletal survey and an isotope bone scan, if possible.

BIOPSY

This is the only definitive way of confirming the diagnosis. It should be performed on the site which is most accessible and will result in least discomfort to the patient. As mentioned above, bone marrow infiltration together with elevated urinary catecholamines may confirm the presence of Stage IV neuroblastoma. If the diagnosis cannot be established by these simple means, biopsy of suspicious lymph nodes or of the primary tumour mass will be required. In the case of the 'blueberry muffin' infant, biopsy of subcutaneous lesions will establish the diagnosis.

URINARY METABOLITES

Increased levels of metabolites of epinephrine, norepinephrine and dopamine are present in approximately 80% of patients with neuroblastoma, and can be measured in urine and serum. Those most commonly measured are 3-methoxy-4-hydroxy-mandelic acid, generally but incorrectly called vanillyl mandelic acid (VMA), total catecholamines, metanephrine and homovanillic acid (HVA). In order to quantitate the urinary excretion of these metabolic products, their levels should be expressed as a total amount per urine volume or, better, as milligram of metabolite per gram of urinary creatinine. Although slight elevations of these metabolites can be found in other tumours, they are most markedly raised in neuroblastoma and phaeochromocytoma.

In the clinical context of the patient's presentation and bone marrow findings, the estimation of the above urinary metabolites is often diagnostic. Furthermore, the level of urinary metabolites can be followed during the course of treatment. In the majority of patients receiving effective therapy, there is a decrease of the excretory products which may fall to normal levels or plateau at an elevated level if there is significant remaining tumour or

Table 19.1 Staging system for neuroblastoma.

Stage I
Tumour confined to organ or structure of origin

Stage II
Tumour extending in continuity beyond the organ or structure of origin, but not crossing the midline. Regional lymph nodes on the homolateral side may be involved

Stage III
Tumour extending in continuity beyond the midline. Regional lymph nodes may be involved bilaterally

Stage IV
Remote disease involving skeleton, organs, soft tissues or distant lymph node groups, etc.

Stage IV-S
Patient who otherwise would be Stage I or II, but who has remote disease confined to liver and/or skin and/or bone marrow (without radiographic evidence of bone involvement)

maturing ganglio neuroma. In patients who relapse, there is often an elevation of the excretory products before there are clinical signs of relapse.

There is growing evidence that the pattern of excretion of urinary catecholamine metabolites may be correlated with prognosis. In patients with Stage III and IV disease, a ratio of VMA/HVA greater than one appears to be associated with greater survival.

Staging

The prognosis given to the parents and the intensity of treatment depends upon the stage of the tumour at presentation. Neuroblastoma is somewhat unique in that both the age and the clinical stage at the time of diagnosis affect prognosis. In general, age and stage go together, with infants having local and resectable tumours and older children, widespread metastatic disease. The most commonly used staging system is that shown in Table 19.1. It should be noted that the IV-S subgroup should be confined to children less than 12 months of age at presentation. The presence of bony metastases signals an almost uniformly fatal outcome.

This staging system applies best to patients with abdominal primaries. For patients with pelvic, thoracic or cervical primaries, it is inappropriate as they usually arise close to and may cross the midline, but are still localized. Tumours in these primary sites should best be considered as local and resectable; regional and unresectable; or metastatic.

Treatment

SURGERY

Complete resection of local tumours is the treatment of choice. This is usually feasible in Stage I and II abdominal primaries and in thoracic and pelvic primaries. Stage III abdominal primaries are rarely resectable because of encroachment on vital structures. Removal of the primary in Stage IV disease at the beginning of treatment does not appear to influence ultimate longterm outcome. The role of delayed primary surgery in Stage IV disease is under investigation.

In patients with spinal cord compression, immediate myelography is mandatory. Neurosurgical decompression will alleviate the immediate clinical problem. Patients with dumbbell lesions can then have the extraspinal component removed as a planned procedure when they have recovered from spinal cord decompression.

IRRADIATION

Although the tumour is relatively sensitive to irradiation, there is no evidence that this modality of treatment has influenced survival. It has no role in the treatment of Stage I or II disease, which is best dealt with surgically.

In Stage III disease, it may be used to attempt local control of irremovable tumour. The dose used varies, 20–30 Gy, with appropriate shielding of vital structures. It is particularly useful in patients with severe bone pain or proptosis where it may provide relief of symptoms in the terminal phase of the illness.

CHEMOTHERAPY

Chemotherapy has made little impact on the ultimate prognosis. Although immediate response rates are encouraging with regression of tumour and clearance of marrow infiltration in 80% of patients, unfortunately, relapse between 6–12 months after the beginning of treatment occurs in the majority of patients. The agents with some demonstrable activity against neuroblastoma are vincristine, cyclophosphamide, VM26, DIC, adriamycin, melphalan and *cis*-platinum. At the present time, there is no substantial evidence that chemotherapy adds to the cure rate of Stage I and II tumours treated with surgery alone. In Stage III and IV disease, combination chemotherapy has been under intensive investigation with disappointing results.

The most commonly used combinations include vincristine and cyclophosphamide; vincristine, cyclophosphamide, adriamycin and DIC; *cis*-platinum and VM26; cyclophosphamide and adriamycin; *cis*-platinum and VM26 followed by high dose melphalan with autologous bone marrow rescue. As with other tumours, any attempts at intensive chemotherapy should only be made in appropriate oncology departments and the parents should be informed of their essentially palliative nature.

In infants with Stage IV-S neuroblastoma, spontaneous remission occurs in 60% of patients without active treatment. The spontaneous remission rate is lower in children over the age of 12 months. In these children, combination chemotherapy with vincristine and cyclophosphamide may accelerate remission.

Prognosis

Tumours arising in the neck, thorax and pelvis are most often Stage I and II and have a good prognosis, while intra-abdominal primaries are most often Stage III and IV and have a poor prognosis.

Two-year survival figures are as follows:

Stage	I	90%
Stage	II	70–80%
Stage	III	20–25%
Stage	IV	10–20%
Stage	IV-S	60–70%

In general, 2 years' survival free of disease is equivalent to cure. However, late recurrences have been reported in adolescence many years after apparently successful initial treatment.

RECOMMENDED READING

ALTMAN A.J. & BAEHNER R.L. (1976) Favorable prognosis for survival in children with coincident opsomyoclonus and neuroblastoma. *Cancer* **37**, 846.

BECKWITH J.B. & MORTIN R.F. (1968) Observations on the histopathology of neuroblastomas. *Journal of Pediatric Surgery* **3**, 106.

BRESLOW N. & MCCANN B. (1971) Statistical estimation of prognosis for children with neuroblastoma. *Cancer Research* **31**, 2098.

EVANS A.E. (ed) (1980) Advances in neuroblastoma research. *Progress in Cancer Research and Therapy* **12**. Raven Press, New York.

EVANS A.E. (1979) Proceedings of the Tumour Board of the Children's Hospital of Philadelphia. IV-S neuroblastoma. *Medical and Pediatric Oncology* **6**, 85.

EVANS A.E., CHATTEN J., D'ANGIO G.J. *et al.* (1980) A review of 17 IV-S neuroblastoma patients at the Children's Hospital of Philadelphia. *Cancer* **45**, 834.

FINKLESTEIN J.Z., KLEMPERER M.R., EVANS A., BERNSTEIN I., LEIKIN S., MCCREADIE S., GROSFIELD J., HITTLE R., WEINER J., SATHER H. & HAMMOND D. (1979) Multiagent chemotherapy for children with metastatic neuroblastoma. *Medical and Pediatric Oncology* **6**, 179.

KING D., GOODMAN J., HAWK T., BOLES E.T. & SAYERS M. (1975) Dumbbell neuroblastomas in children. *Archives of Surgery* **110**, 888.

JAFFE N. (1976) Neuroblastoma: Review of the literature and an examination of factors contributing to its enigmatic character. *Cancer Treatment Reviews* **3**, 61.

NECHELLES T.F., RAUSEN A.R., KUNG F.H. & POCHEDLY C. (1978) Immunotherapy in advanced neuroblastoma. *Cancer* **41**, 1282.

PUNT J., PRITCHARD J., PINCOTT J.R. & TILL K. (1980) Neuroblastoma: A review of 21 cases presenting with spinal cord compression. *Cancer* **45**, 3095.

Chapter 20
Soft Tissue Sarcomas

Apart from rhabdomyosarcoma, soft tissue sarcomas are rare tumours in children. They have a common characteristic of a tendency to local recurrence. Early metastatic spread is a prominent feature of rhabdomyosarcoma, while other types may metastasize late.

RHABDOMYOSARCOMA

Incidence

This tumour represents 4–8% of malignancies under the age of 15 years and occurs most commonly in children under 7 years of age. As rhabdomyosarcoma may occur anywhere in the body, the presenting signs and symptoms vary according to the primary site. The intergroup rhabdomyosarcoma studies from the USA show that orbit and head and neck tumours account for 36%, extremities 23%, genitourinary 18% and trunk 8%, of all tumours.

Presentation

Orbital tumours are usually detected early because of their site and are invariably localized.

Nasopharyngeal and paranasal sinus primaries present with nasal obstruction, epistaxis, dysphagia, nasal discharge and sinusitis. A pharyngeal mass may be present or extension into the nares may occur.

Middle ear tumours present with discharge, pain, chronic otitis media and, occasionally, a polypoid mass in the external auditory canal.

Retroperitoneal tumours may reach a very large size before they cause symptoms. Local infiltration is usually widespread. Abdominal pain, a mass, or obstruction of the gastrointestinal or genitourinary tract are the usual presenting features.

Genitourinary tract interference with bladder or bowel function is the usual method of presentation. The typical sarcoma botryoides protruding from the introitus is only occasionally seen and is most common in girls. Paratesticular rhabdomyosarcoma usually presents as a unilateral, painless movable intrascrotal swelling which may transilluminate if a hydrocoele is also present. Perineal and anal lesions usually present with local swelling which may be confused with an abscess.

Metastatic disease

Metastatic disease at the time of presentation occurs in approximately 20% of patients. Most commonly, it involves lungs, lymph nodes, bones, bone marrow, liver and brain. One rare but important mode of presentation of metastatic disease is sudden onset of paraplegia. In such patients, emergency laminectomy is required before the definitive diagnosis is established. Neuroblastoma and non-Hodgkin's lymphoma are more common neoplastic causes of sudden onset of paraplegia.

Truncal and extremity tumours usually present as a local swelling which has been present for a considerable length of time before presentation. There may be associated pain and some local erythema. Not infrequently, the lesion has been mistaken for cellulitis or chronic abscess and treated with antibiotics. Occasionally, extremity lesions may be calcified. Truncal lesions may present with extensions to the pleural or peritoneal cavities, in which case the child may have symptoms and signs of pleural effusion or ascites.

Pathology

Apart from the characteristic grape-like clusters of sarcoma botryoides, the macroscopic appearance is not characteristic. Rhabdomyosarcoma usually deeply infiltrates surrounding structures. Microscopically, four categories are recognized: embryonal botryoid, embryonal, alveolar and pleomorphic. In children, the embryonal type is commonest. Embryonal tumours have a better prognosis than the alveolar type. The majority of patients with head and neck, orbital or genitourinary tumours (70%) have embryonal histology, while extremity and trunk lesions are most often alveolar (40–50%). There is a group of tumours with undifferentiated histology. These constitute some 16% of patients.

In some, histological features are suggestive of Ewing's sarcoma (see Chapter 21) while, in others, the diagnosis of rhabdomyosarcoma is made by exclusion.

Staging

Full clinical staging should be performed before biopsy and/or removal of the primary lesion. This involves chest X-ray, bone scan and/or skeletal survey, CAT scans, bone marrow aspiration and baseline biochemistry. CSF examination and CAT scan of the cranial fossa and brain should be performed in patients with parameningeal primaries.

Whenever possible, the initial biopsy should be a wide local excision. In some situations, however, such as facial or perineal primaries, a needle biopsy may be the first step in diagnosis. This also applies to sites where excisional biopsy would be unnecessarily mutilating. The US Intergroup Rhabdomyosarcoma Study suggests the following staging system given in Table 20.1.

Treatment

Prior to the development of effective multimodal therapy, the survival rate of patients with rhabdomyosarcoma was in the range 12–30%. With the demonstration that the tumour was sensitive to irradiation and chemotherapy, much improved results are now obtained, with disease-free survival rates of at least 60% at 5 years. Each of the three separate treatment modalities will be considered individually.

SURGERY

Biopsy is obviously essential for diagnosis and, whenever possible, should be excisional as, for example, in a lesion of the extremity, where wide local excision is possible. For head and neck primaries, biopsy only is indicated in view of the significant cosmetic and functional deformity that could be involved in total surgical excision.

Chemotherapy and/or irradiation may convert a previously inoperable tumour into an operable one. This is especially important in genitourinary primaries where preliminary chemotherapy and/or radiotherapy may shrink the tumour to a size that makes local resection feasible without recourse to mutilating surgery, e.g. pelvic exenteration.

Table 20.1 Staging system for rhabdomyosarcoma.

Group I
Localized disease completely resected

Group II
Localized disease, microscopic residual
(a) Grossly resected tumour with microscopic residual. No evidence of regional node involvement
(b) Regional disease, completely resected. No known microscopic residual disease
(c) Regional disease with involved nodes grossly resected, but with evidence of microscopic residual disease

Group III
Incomplete resection or biopsy with gross residual disease

Group IV
Distant metastatic disease present at diagnosis.

o

IRRADIATION THERAPY

The usual dose is 50 Gy given in equal fractions over 5 weeks.

The US Intergroup Rhabdomyosarcoma Study has shown that for patients in Group I, postoperative irradiation therapy can be safely omitted without compromising local control, provided adequate adjuvant chemotherapy is given. Similarly, in Group II, III and IV patients, local control has not been compromised by delaying irradiation therapy for 6 weeks, while intensive chemotherapy is given to control both local and metastatic disease. Spinal irradiation is reserved for parameningeal primaries (nasopharynx, middle ear, mastoid, paranasal sinus, pterygopalatine infratemporal fossa) which show definite intraspinal extension on radiological investigations or tumour cells in the CSF.

CHEMOTHERAPY

The VAC programme (vincristine, actinomycin D and cyclophosphamide), in one of its many variations, can be considered as standard. In patients with Stage III and IV disease, the role of adriamycin in addition to VAC is being explored in an attempt to improve long-term survival. Adjuvant chemotherapy is usually given (empirically) for 2 years from the time of diagnosis. The details of the VAC regimen can be obtained from the Rhabdomyosarcoma Intergroup Study protocol. It should be administered only in haematology/oncology centres. The usual regimens consist of:

Vincristine 1.5 mg/m^2 (maximum dose 2 mg)

Actinomycin D 1.5 mg/m^2 and cyclophosphamide given i.v. every 3 weeks.

In Stage III and IV disease adriamycin 40 mg/m^2 alternates with actinomycin D.

Prognosis

Prognosis is related to age, clinical grouping, site of presentation and tumour histology. Based on the Intergroup Rhabdomyosarcoma Study I, children between the ages of 2–6 years have a better survival rate than those aged 11–15 years. Orbital and genitourinary tumours have the best survival probability (75–80%); non-orbital head and neck and trunk intermediate (50–60%); and extremities and retroperitoneal the worst (20–40%). Botryoid embryonal tumours have the best (70%); solid embryonal intermediate (65%); and alveolar or pleomorphic the worst (20–30%) survival probability. The estimated probability of survival according to clinical grouping is:

Group I	90%
Group II	80%
Group III	60%
Group IV	10%

In patients with parameningeal lesions, it was initially reported that 30% developed meningeal extensions of tumour. However, in the Intergroup Rhabdomyosarcoma Study II, a follow-up of 12 patients considered to be at high risk of meningeal disease and not given spinal irradiation, none developed meningeal spread. This suggests that 'prophylactic' craniospinal irradiation is unnecessary.

FIBROSARCOMA

Fibrosarcoma is rare in childhood and is characterized by a tendency to local recurrence. Most arise in the limbs. Difficulty may be encountered by the pathologist in determining whether the lesion is benign or malignant.

The treatment of choice is wide local excision followed by irradiation therapy. If local recurrence occurs, amputation is indicated. Preoperative irradiation may convert a marginally operable lesion into an operable one. Metastases occur uncommonly, but may occur late.

Because of the rarity of this tumour, the role of adjuvant chemotherapy is difficult to assess. Patients with metastatic disease will usually respond to chemotherapy but this is unfortunately, usually only shortlived. Active agents are adriamycin and DIC (see Synovial Sarcoma below), with VAC programmes being also effective.

SYNOVIAL SARCOMA

Synovial sarcoma usually presents as a painless mass in the extremities. Its main characteristics are local recurrence and pulmonary metastases whose appearance may be delayed for some years.

Amputation offers the best prospect of cure. Wide local excision, followed by irradiation therapy, may be a satisfactory alternative. Again, the precise role of adjuvant chemotherapy has yet to be determined.

RECOMMENDED READING

Rhabdomyosarcoma

Dritschillo A., Weichselbaum R., Cassady J.R., Jaffe N., Green D. & Filler R.M. (1978) The role of radiation therapy in the treatment of soft tissue sarcomas of childhood. *Cancer* **42**, 1192.

Maurer H.M., Moon T., Donaldson M., Fernandez C., Gehan E.A., Hammond D., Hays D.M., Lawrence W., Newton W., Ragab A., Raney B., Soule E., Sutow W.W. & Tefft M. (1977) The Intergroup Rhabdomyosarcoma Study. A preliminary report. *Cancer* **40**, 2015.

Raney R.B., Hays D.M., Lawrence W., *et al.* (1978) Paratesticular rhabdomyosarcoma in childhood. *Cancer* **42**, 729.

RIVARD G., ORTEGA J., HITTLE R., NITSCHKE R. & KARON M. (1975) Intensive chemotherapy as primary treatment for rhabdomyosarcoma of the pelvis. *Cancer* **36**, 1593.

TEFFT M., FERNANDEZ C.H. & MOON T.E. (1977) Rhabdomyosarcoma: Response with chemotherapy prior to radiation in patients with gross residual disease. *Cancer* **39**, 665.

TEFFT M., FERNANDEZ C., DONALDSON M., NEWTON W. & MOON T.E. (1978) Incidence of meningeal involvement by rhabdomyosarcoma of the head and neck in children. A report of the Intergroup Rhabdomyosarcoma Study. *Cancer* **42**, 253.

Fibrosarcoma

SOULE E.H. & PRITCHARD D.J. (1977) Fibrosarcoma in infants and children. A review of 110 cases. *Cancer* **40**, 1711.

WILBUR J.R., SUTOW W.W., SULLIVAN M.P. & GOTTLIEB J.A. (1975) Chemotherapy of sarcomas. *Cancer* **36**, 765.

Synovial sarcoma

SHIU M.H., MCCORMACK P.M., HAJDU S.I. & FORTNER J.G. (1979) Surgical treatment of tenosynovial sarcoma. *Cancer* **43**, 889.

Chapter 21
Bone Tumours

General features

Ewing's sarcoma and osteosarcoma are the commonest primary bone tumours and account for 10–12% of childhood malignancies. These tumours are sometimes a diagnostic challenge, and always a therapeutic one. Their treatment may involve mutilative procedures such as amputation and, in addition, the complications of intensive irradiation and chemotherapy. These tumours occur predominantly in teenage and adolescence, further magnifying the difficulties of treatment. The management of such patients should only be undertaken in specialized units that can provide and coordinate early and effective limb prosthesis, psychological and social support, as well as expert medical and surgical treatment.

There are other less common primary bone tumours which are rarely confused with Ewing's and osteosarcoma. These include non-Hodgkin's lymphoma of bone, fibrosarcoma, chondrosarcoma and chordoma. Metastatic bone tumours are also seldom confused with primary bone tumours as there is usually evidence of the primary lesion. The more important metastatic tumours include neuroblastoma, rhabdomyosarcoma, retinoblastoma and Wilms' tumour.

A number of non-malignant conditions should be considered in the differential diagnosis of primary bone tumours. The most important ones are osteomyelitis, simple bone cysts, aneurysmal bone cysts, dysplasias, osteoid osteoma and benign osteoblastomas.

OSTEOSARCOMA

Incidence and clinical features

Osteosarcoma affects boys more often than girls, with a peak incidence between ages 10–25 years. Ninety per cent arise in long bones, with the lower end of femur and upper end of tibia accounting for at least 50%.

Patients usually present with pain followed by swelling of the affected region. A pathological fracture is occasionally the presenting finding and occasionally the patient may be febrile, raising the possibility of osteomyelitis. Radiological investigations are most helpful. Typical findings include destruction of bone, formation of bone within the tumour, soft tissue mass extending from the surface of the affected bone and reactive periosteal new bone. A bone scan is essential to exclude or delineate bone metastases. In addition to a chest X-ray, a CAT scan of the lungs should be performed to diagnose or exclude pulmonary metastatic lesions. The serum alkaline phosphatase is elevated, but does not correlate with prognosis.

Pathology

Histological sections show abnormal osteoid formed by tumour cells and closely related to them. Nuclear pleomorphism is a characteristic feature. Giant atypical mitotic figures and multinucleated tumour giant cells are also quite common. A number of histological sub-types have been described including the paraosteal, periosteal and a tumour which is extremely vascular and is known as telangiectatic osteosarcoma, which must be distinguished from aneurysmal bone cysts.

Treatment

SURGERY

Until recently, immediate amputation was the treatment of choice. More recently, limb preservation has been undertaken as definitive surgical treatment. *En bloc* resection is only undertaken after intensive preoperative chemotherapy when there is clinical and radiologic evidence of tumour shrinkage in response to the chemotherapy. The presence of pulmonary metastases is not considered a contraindication to *en bloc* resection. Such procedures have been performed on the distal femur, shoulder girdle, proximal tibia and the fibula. Preoperative angiography is required to ensure that neurovascular bundles are not involved by the tumour. When amputation is undertaken, immediate fitting of a prosthesis is desirable to improve both the physical and psychological rehabilitation of the patient.

Excision of solitary pulmonary metastases has been undertaken for many years before there was any form of effective chemotherapy, with six of 22 patients thus treated reported alive at 5 years. With the evolvement of effective chemotherapy, resection of pulmonary metastases has been undertaken, even in the presence of multiple and bilateral lesions. In some units, surgery has been accompanied by intensive chemotherapy, while in others no chemotherapy has been given. Thoracotomies have been performed on multiple occasions. Preliminary results using both approaches to treatment suggest a 30% 3 year survival.

IRRADIATION

Although irradiation may have to be used in patients with non-resectable primary tumours (vertebral column, skull), it is mainly reserved for the treatment of painful bony or pleural metastases. The role of bilateral 'prophylactic' pulmonary irradiation is under investigation but, so far, results are only preliminary. Irradiation of pulmonary metastases has also been used in conjunction with surgery and chemotherapy, but results appear to be no better than those obtained with surgery and chemotherapy, or surgery alone.

CHEMOTHERAPY

This remains a controversial area. Early reports of successful use of high dose methotrexate with citrovorum factor rescue from the Sidney Farber Cancer Centre established the value of chemotherapy in the treatment of this tumour when compared with historical controls. Similarly, the South Western Oncology Group showed that intensive multiple agent chemotherapy (acronym, Conpadri I) was also effective in prolonging disease-free survival when compared with historical controls. As a result of these studies, there has been further intensification of chemotherapy in many centres with the use of very large doses of methotrexate with citrovorum rescue combined with multiple agents (T_7 and T_{10} protocols, Sloan Kettering Memorial Hospital) or with vincristine and adriamycin. In other centres, investigators were not convinced that it was necessary to use very high doses of methotrexate and patients have been randomized to adjuvant chemotherapy programmes, comparing intermediate dose methotrexate with high dose regimens.

The situation has been further confused by reports emanating from the Mayo Clinic that, in patients treated with amputation alone, the long-term disease-free survival rates were approximately 50% rather than the 20% quoted in historical controls. Preliminary reports of a randomized trial comparing chemotherapy with methotrexate and vincristine versus no chemotherapy are reported to show no significant difference between the two groups.

Because of the confused state of chemotherapy in this tumour, only tentative recommendations can be made. It is a fact that the majority of specialized units use adjuvant chemotherapy consisting of intermediate or high dose methotrexate and other agents, most commonly vincristine and adriamycin. Most centres that use such chemotherapy programmes report a 50–60% disease-free rate with a median follow-up which varies between 2–7 years. If limb preservation is to be used, then the best results are reported with preoperative chemotherapy using multiple agents and very large doses of methotrexate. It is the author's opinion that those units not using adjuvant chemotherapy will have to conclusively prove that in unselected patients, the results of surgery alone are as good as those with adjuvant chemotherapy.

Until such times as this proof appears, there appear to be valid grounds for the use of chemotherapy. In patients with metastatic disease, alternating courses of *cis*-platinum and high dose methotrexate with citrovorum factor rescue have been associated with tumour response which has permitted surgical excision of the pulmonary lesions.

EWING'S SARCOMA

Incidence and clinical features

The disease occurs at a slightly earlier age than osteosarcoma and is more common in males than in females. Unlike osteosarcoma, Ewing's sarcoma is extremely rare in blacks.

From data available from the Intergroup Ewing's Sarcoma Study I, the primary tumours occur most commonly in lower extremities (43%), axial skeleton (21%), pelvis (18%), upper extremities (12%) and shoulder (5%).

The presenting features are usually a painless swelling which, not infrequently, has been present for a considerable time. In a significant number of patients, there are also symptoms of intermittent fever, malaise and weight loss. These children are often misdiagnosed as having osteomyelitis, and the true diagnosis may only be established when antibiotics have failed to control the disease and a second biopsy is undertaken. An uncommon but important mode of presentation is that with spinal cord compression from Ewing's sarcoma originating from the vertebral column. In these patients, emergency decompression of the spinal cord must be undertaken before a definitive diagnosis is established.

Radiological investigations are most helpful. Plain X-rays classically show bony changes consisting of a combination of destruction and sclerosis surrounded by multiple layers of periosteal new bone; so called 'onion skin' layers. A 'sunray' appearance is seen when the tumour has broken through the periosteum. Plain X-rays of the chest, radioisotope bone scan and bone marrow aspirates are mandatory, as 20% of patients present with metastatic lesions to bone and lung.

For purposes of defining the field of irradiation, a CAT scan of the tumour can be most helpful. CAT scans of lungs may be performed as a routine investigation or when there is suspicion or evidence of pulmonary metastases. In the case of spinal Ewing's, CAT scans of spine and myelography are required. Of the usual blood tests, the ESR and serum lactic dehydrogenase levels are most useful. The ESR is often markedly elevated, helping to distinguish Ewing's sarcoma from osteomyelitis. Lactic dehydrogenase levels may also be elevated and raised levels appear to be associated with a worse response to treatment.

Pathology

The most common histological appearance consists of structureless sheets of rather uniform, darkly staining tumour cells. New bone formation does not occur within the tumour but, if present, is invariably beneath the periosteum. A filigree pattern consisting of elevated fibrovascular septa arranged around complex, often bilateral strands of tumour cells, is a distinct variant. Organization into lobules and pseudorosettes is not uncommon. Pseudorosettes are distinguished from neuroblastoma by the absence of neurofibrillary material.

In the course of the Intergroup Rhabdomyosarcoma Study, an extraskeletal variety of Ewing's sarcoma has been described. These tumours appear to arise from soft tissue rather than bone. There appear to be two histological types, one with typical bony Ewing's sarcoma called Type I, and the other in which the cells are larger, more irregular and have less dense chromatin (Type II). Patients with this type of tumour appear to respond well to treatment.

Treatment

Ewing's sarcoma metastasizes frequently, and despite the fact that it is radiosensitive, cure of local disease can only be achieved using high doses of irradiation. This results in one of the major dilemmas of the treatment of Ewing's sarcoma, namely, how to control primary disease without causing long-term unacceptable toxicity to growing bone and surrounding vital tissues.

SURGERY

Biopsy is essential for diagnosis. When performing a biopsy, a limited amount of bony tissue should be taken from bones that may subsequently be irradiated, as there may be poor healing of the biopsy site in irradiated bone and consequent pathological fractures.

Retrospective analyses of results of treatment from the Mayo Clinic indicate that long-term disease-free survival rates are improved by surgical resection. There is also convincing evidence that local recurrence rates are as high as 20%, particularly in the humerus and pelvis, when the dose of local irradiation must be reduced below 60 Gy for fear of damage to vital surrounding tissue. This is particularly important when the site of origin is in the pelvis, chest wall, skull or spine, where toxicity to bladder, myocardium and lungs, eyes and mucous membranes and spinal cord, respectively, limit the dose of irradiation. In such sites, immediate *en bloc* excision of tumours may appear desirable, but as Ewing's sarcoma is a locally infiltrative lesion, resection must be delayed until local shrinkage of tumour is obtained with chemotherapy and/or irradiation.

In lesions of the extremities, excision of expendable bones such as the fibula reduces the risks of local recurrence and may eliminate the need for irradiation or permit the use of low dose irradiation only. When lesions arise from major bones, e.g. femur and tibia, amputation is usually not performed as the initial form of treatment because there is a 40–50% chance that despite adjuvant chemotherapy, distant metastases will develop in other bones or the lungs. However, the long-term effects of irradiation, which cause unacceptable shortening of the limb, pathological fractures or lymphoedema or the fear of local recurrence, may force delayed amputation.

IRRADIATION

Irradiation rapidly resolves pain and reduces the size of the tumour. To reduce local recurrence rates to below 10%, tumour doses of at least 55–60 Gy are required. As mentioned above, this is usually not possible with axial lesions. The whole of the soft tissue component and the whole of the involved bone are treated initially to a dose of 45–50 Gy. In extremity lesions, a strip of skin and subcutaneous tissue should be shielded to prevent circumferential fibrosis and the later development of lymphoedema. If possible, once the initial dose is given, the field is decreased to cover the tumour with a 3–5 cm margin and a further 10–15 Gy are given to this area. Other experimental approaches include prophylactic bilateral pulmonary irradiation to a total dose of 15–18 Gy.

In children, such aggressive irradiation is associated with potentially severe long-term morbidity, e.g. epiphyseal arrest leading to growth failure, fibrosis, muscle atrophy, contracture and pathological fractures and induction of second tumours.

In patients with metastatic pulmonary disease at the time of presentation, lung field irradiation is necessary as part of primary treatment. In this situation, the whole of both lungs are irradiated to a total dose of 15–18 Gy. In patients who relapse during treatment, palliative irradiation may be given to sites of recurrence. A more intensive approach is now under investigation using sequential hemibody irradiation. The upper half of the body is irradiated to 5 Gy after the first course of chemotherapy. After a 6 week rest, the lower half is irradiated with the same dose.

CHEMOTHERAPY

Adjuvant combination chemotherapy significantly increases the proportion of disease-free patients at 2 and 5 years. Before the use of chemotherapy, the 2 year survival was 25%, and 5 year less than 10%. Combinations of vincristine, actinomycin D, cyclophosphamide and adriamycin have been most successful, resulting in median disease-free survival times of 237 plus weeks. The results achieved with vincristine, cyclophosphamide and actinomycin D alone are significantly worse than when adriamycin is also used.

If metastatic disease is present at the time of diagnosis, a similar regimen may be employed. If metastases appear during treatment, a number of intensive chemotherapeutic regimens are under investigation. These include the combined use of 5-fluorouracil, VM26 and BCNU or combinations of VM26 and *cis*-platinum

Care must be taken to avoid the combined toxicity of chemotherapy and irradiation therapy. If the pelvis is being irradiated, then cyclophosphamide should be deferred until irradiation is finished because of the combined toxic effects on the bladder mucosa. Actinomycin D should also be delayed if the mucosa of the mouth, nasopharynx, large areas of the gastrointestinal tract or lungs are in the field. If the chest wall has been irradiated, the total dose of adriamycin should be below 300 mg/m^2, as the combined cardiotoxicity of heart irradiation and adriamycin are cumulative.

Prognosis

Based on the results of the Intergroup Ewing's Sarcoma Study I, certain clinical features as well as the site of origin correlate with prognosis. Females appear to have a better survival rate, and patients in the 11–15 year age group seem to respond better than those under 10 or over 16 years. Patients with duration of symptoms of less than 1 month have a superior disease-free survival compared to those with symptom duration of more than 1 month. The most favourable sites are distal limb or extraskeletal (77% disease-free at 2 years), sternum, clavicle, skull and vertebrae (68% disease-free at 2 years), followed by proximal limb and ribs (50% disease-free at 2 years). The least favourable site is pelvic, with only 40% of patients disease-free at 2 years.

RECOMMENDED READING

Osteosarcoma

BURGERS J.M.V., BREUER K., DOBBENBURG VAN O.A., HAZEBROEK F., VAS A. & VOUTE P.A. (1980) Role of metastectomy without chemotherapy in the management of osteosarcoma in children. *Cancer* **45**, 1664.

CORTES E.P., HOLLAND J.E., WANG J.J., SINKS L.F., BLOM J., SENN H., BANK A. & GLIDEWELL O. (1974) Amputation and adriamycin in primary osteosarcoma. *New England Journal of Medicine* **291**, 998.

EDMONSON J.H., GREEN S.J., IVINS J.C., GILCHRIST G.S., *et al.* (1980) Methotrexate as adjuvant treatment for primary osteosarcoma. *New England Journal of Medicine* **303**, 642.

FARR G.H., HUVOS A.G., MARCOVE R.C., HIGINBOTHAM N.L. & FOOTE JR. F.W. (1974) Telangiectatic osteogenic sarcoma. A review of twenty-eight cases. *Cancer* **34**, 1150.

JAFFE N., FREI III E., TRAGGIS D. & BISHOP Y. (1974) Adjuvant methotrexate and citrovorum-factor treatment of osteogenic sarcoma. *New England Journal of Medicine* **291**, 994.

ROSEN G., MURPHY L.M., HUVOS A.G., GUTIERREZ M. & MARCOVE R.C. (1976) Chemotherapy en bloc resection and prosthetic bone replacement in the treatment of osteogenic sarcoma. *Cancer* **37**, 1.

ROSEN G., HUVOS A.G., MOSENDE C., *et al.* (1978) Chemotherapy and thoracotomy for metastatic osteogenic sarcoma. A model for adjuvant chemotherapy and the rationale for the timing of thoracic surgery. *Cancer* **41**, 841.

ROSEN G., MARCOVE R.C., CAPARROS B., NIRENBERG A., KOSLOFF C. & HUVOS A.G. (1979) Primary osteogenic sarcoma. The rationale for preoperative chemotherapy and delayed surgery. *Cancer* **43**, 2163.

SUTOW W., GEHAN E.A., VIETTI T.J., FRIAS E.A. & DYMENT P.G. (1976) Multidrug chemotherapy in primary treatment of osteosarcoma. *Journal Bone and Joint Surgery* **58A**, 629.

SUTOW W.W. (1978) Primary adjuvant chemotherapy in osteosarcoma. *The Cancer Bulletin* **30**, 178.

YUNIS E.J. (1979) Prognostic factors in osteosarcoma. *Cancer* **36**, 2179.

Ewing's sarcoma

CHAN R.C., SUTOW W.W., LINDBERG R.D., SAMUELS M.L., MURRAY J.A. & JOHNSTON D.A. (1979) Management and results of localized Ewing's sarcoma. *Cancer* **43**, 1001.

GRAHAM-POLE J. (1979) Ewing's sarcoma: Treatment with high dose radiation and adjuvant chemotherapy. *Medical and Pediatric Oncology* 7, 1.

GLICKMAN A.S., MAURER H.M. & VIETTI T.J. (1979) Overview of conferences on sarcomas of soft tissue and bone in childhood. *Medical and Pediatric Oncology* 7, 55.

LE MEVEL B.P., HOERNI B., DURANT D., *et al.* (1979) EORTC/GTO Adjuvant chemotherapy program for primary Ewing's sarcoma: Results at 5 years. *Recent Results in Cancer Research* **68**, 52.

PEREZ C.A., RAZEK A., TEFFT M., NESBIT M., BURGERT O.E., KISSANE J., VIETTI T. & GEHAN E.A. (1977) Analysis of local tumour control in Ewing's sarcoma. Preliminary results of a co-operative intergroup study. *Cancer* **40**, 2864.

POMEROY T.C. & JOHNSON R.E. (1975) Combined modality therapy of Ewing's sarcoma. *Cancer* **35**, 36.

ROSEN G., CAPARROS B., MOSENDE C., MCCORMICK B., HUVOS A. & MARCOVE R.C. (1978) Curability of Ewing's sarcoma and considerations for future therapeutic trials. *Cancer* **41**, 888.

SOULE E.H., NEWTON JR. W., MOON T.E. & TEFFT M. (1978) Extraskeletal Ewing's sarcoma. *Cancer* **42**, 259.

TEFFT M., LATTIN P.B., JEREB B. *et al.* (1976) Treatment of rhabdomyosarcoma and Ewing's sarcoma of childhood: Acute and late effects on normal tissue following combination therapy with emphasis on the role of irradiation combined with chemotherapy. *Cancer* **37**, 1201.

TEFFT M., CHABORA B.M. & ROSEN G. (1977) Radiation in bone sarcomas — a re-evaluation in the era of intensive systemic chemotherapy. *Cancer* **39**, 424.

Chapter 22
Primary Central Nervous System Tumours

Primary CNS tumours are second only to leukaemia as a cause of malignancy and death in children with tumours. CNS tumours occur at any age, with a peak incidence between 5 and 10 years. Boys are affected more often than girls. In contradistinction to adults, about 60% are infratentorial. Few centres have approached the treatment of CNS tumours with the combined approach practised in other solid tumours of childhood. Standard treatment for CNS tumours currently consists of surgery, wherever feasible, followed by irradiation therapy. The role of adjuvant chemotherapy is uncertain at the present time. The existence of the blood-brain barrier has been considered to be the main stumbling block in devising effective chemotherapy for brain tumours. However, the blood-brain barrier may not be wholly intact in brain tumours and can in part be overcome by selecting lipid soluble chemotherapeutic agents or increasing serum concentrations of water soluble drugs to levels which allow them to enter the CNS, e.g. the use of high dose methotrexate with folinic acid rescue in presymptomatic treatment of CNS leukaemia.

Pathology and classification

There is a lack of agreement amongst pathologists as to nomenclature and classification of primary CNS tumours. A simplified working classification is shown in Table 22.1.

Presenting symptoms

These vary immensely depending upon the age of the patient, location of the tumour and its rate of growth. Briefly, they are usually as follows:

1 Raised intracranial pressure producing symptoms such as headaches, vomiting, change in personality and regression of skills, and signs such as papilloedema, enlargement of the head and ataxia.

2 Cranial nerve palsies. A squint in a child over 2 years calls for intensive investigations.

3 Endocrine disturbance with delayed growth; diabetes insipidus; precocious sexual development.

4 Focal neurological signs usually appear late, except in brain stem gliomas.
5 Epilepsy occurs in up to 25% of patients.

Investigations

Standard skull X-ray may show split sutures, bony erosion or increased digital markings. Tumour calcification is uncommon. Pneumoencephalography may demonstrate abnormalities of the ventricular system. CSF can be

Table 22.1 Simple classification of CNS tumours.

1 *Tumours showing glial differentiation*
Astrocytoma
(a) well differentiated
(b) with anaplasia
Ependymoma
(a) papillary
(b) non-papillary
(c) poorly differentiated
Oligodendroglioma

2 *Tumours of primitive embryonal or undifferentiated cells*
Medulloblastoma

3 *Germ cell tumours*
Germinoma

4 *Tumours of choroid plexus*
Papilloma
Carcinoma

5 *Craniopharyngiomas*

6 *Teratomas*

7 *Tumours of nerves*
Neurofibroma
Neurilemmona
Optic nerve glioma

8 *Tumours of the meninges*
Meningioma
Meningiosarcoma

9 *Tumours of vascular tissue*
Haemangioglioblastoma
Haemangioma
Haemangiosarcoma

10 *Metastatic tumours*

obtained at this time, obviating the need for lumbar puncture with its attendant dangers. Elevated CSF protein is highly suggestive of a tumour. The presence of malignant cells is of course diagnostic.

Arteriography may aid in localizing the tumour and delineating its extent. Isotope brain scans are of particular value in delineating supratentorial tumours and are complementary to arteriography.

Most of the above investigations have been supplanted to a large extent by the newer technique of computerized axial tomography (CAT). This is a non-invasive technique whose only drawback is that general anaesthesia is needed in children who are unable to lie still. From the amount of information available from CAT scanning, it should be considered as a first line investigation in a child with a suspected brain tumour.

Treatment

SURGERY

Obviously, total removal of the tumour is the procedure of choice. This is rarely possible in CNS tumours because of their location and the resultant severe neurological defect that may follow total excision. An Ommaya reservoir or ventriculoperitoneal or ventriculoatrial shunt may be inserted if the symptoms of raised intracranial pressure require early alleviation.

Macroscopically, complete removal of medulloblastoma and ependymoma is usually feasible, but microscopic residual disease is nearly always left behind. In contradistinction, brain stem gliomas and tumours of the pineal region are inoperable because of their close association with vital areas of the brain. Here, diagnosis is often made on clinical and neuroradiological grounds alone. Surgical exploration is sometimes worthwhile, as a small biopsy is occasionally feasible or a cystic element may be present which can be removed.

As complete removal as possible is the aim of surgery for supratentorial tumours, depending upon their size and location. The cystic element of cystic astrocytomas is usually completely removable, although the tumour nodule itself may be irremovable.

IRRADIATION THERAPY

Radiotherapeutic techniques vary according to the histological type of tumour. Improved radiotherapy techniques and equipment have been responsible for the early improvement in survival of children with brain tumours.

Medulloblastomas and ependymomas are treated with whole neuraxis irradiation. The tumour dose is 45–50 Gy, with 40 Gy to the spinal theca. Treatment is given over a 4–6 week period.

Astrocytomas are treated with a tumour dose of 45 Gy over 4–6 weeks. The tumour bed, plus a wide margin of normal brain, is treated. Low grade and cystic astrocytomas often do not require treatment with irradiation therapy.

Brain stem gliomas are treated to a total dose of 45–50 Gy over a 4–6 weeks' period. The tumour bed, together with a wide area of normal brain and the upper two cervical spinal cord segments, are treated.

Choroid plexus tumours not totally removed, require postoperative irradiation. Pineal tumours are usually radiosensitive, but require neuraxis irradiation.

In general, irradiation therapy should commence within 2 weeks of surgery, provided the patient's clinical condition is satisfactory. Dexamethasone, which has usually been commenced prior to, or subsequent to, surgery, should be continued for the duration of the irradiation therapy. It should then be tapered to zero if the patient's clinical condition will allow. In this way, a baseline clinical assessment can be made against which future progress can be assessed, especially if chemotherapy is to be used.

CHEMOTHERAPY

The major success of adjuvant chemotherapy in other paediatric tumours has been in the eradication of micrometastases. The situation in CNS tumours is obviously different. For chemotherapeutic agents to be effective in CNS tumours, their prime effect must be on the growth of the primary tumour, while the eradication of micrometastases is of little importance.

As previously discussed, the major problem in chemotherapy is the blood-brain barrier. For this reason, most of the chemotherapeutic regimens have used lipid soluble drugs such as the nitrosoureas. A list of the more common single agents that have been tested in brain tumours is shown in Table 22.2 The importance of the blood-brain barrier is called into question by the findings of van Eys and colleagues who showed that MOPP chemotherapy, which consists of water soluble drugs, can reduce in size recurrent CNS tumours. This raises the question of the intactness of the blood-brain barrier when the CNS has been previously irradiated. The findings of van Eys have been confirmed by others and are supported by experimental evidence of the disruption of the blood-brain barrier following CNS irradiation in acute lymphocytic leukaemia.

Table 22.2 Chemotherapeutic agents used in CNS tumours.

Drugs	Response rate (%)
BCNU	30–40
CCNU	30–40
Me CCNU	30–40
Vincristine	30
Procarbazine	30–40
Epipodophyllotoxin VM26	30
Methotrexate	30
Bleomycin	–
Mithramycin	–
DIC	–

Most current brain tumour protocols employ a combination of vincristine, procarbazine and/or a nitrosourea. Methotrexate, although active, can produce leucoencephalopathy in children who have also received irradiation therapy, and so its use is strictly limited.

Medulloblastoma shows the best response to chemotherapy, with complete remission having been achieved in a significant number of children with recurrent disease. The duration of these is, unfortunately, short; approximately 9 months. The role of chemotherapy in an adjuvant setting has yet to be definitively delineated. There is growing evidence from European and USA studies that adjuvant chemotherapy reduces the incidence of late CNS relapses.

Currently available chemotherapeutic agents would seem to have little role to play in the treatment of brain stem gliomas. Some responses have been achieved, but, again, invariably of short duration only. Currently available agents are unlikely to be helpful and new agents will have to be discovered.

A more fruitful approach may be the development of radiosensitizers, such as metronidazole, 5-fluorouracil and hydroxyurea. As radioresistance is one cause of treatment failure, radiosensitizers may enhance the effect of irradiation therapy and lead to improved tumour control. Studies are also needed on the use of radiosensitizers combined with adjuvant chemotherapy.

Myelosuppression is an important side-effect of many of these regimens and is likely to be more marked in children with complete neuraxis irradiation. Chronic myelosuppression, especially thrombocytopenia, may be seen in patients who have had long courses of the nitrosoureas, and this may limit both dose and number of courses of therapy given.

Prognosis

Survival figures for primary CNS tumours represent those achieved with surgery and irradiation therapy. Representative figures are given below. As mentioned earlier, whether the administration of adjuvant chemotherapy will lead to an improvement in prognosis, remains to be proven. Controlled clinical trials are the only way of answering this question.

For medulloblastoma, typical survival figures are:

2 years	50%
5 years	35–40%
10 years	25–30%

For patients with ependymomas, survival varies with the histological grade of malignancy. With low grade tumours, 5 year survival rates of 80% have been achieved. The prognosis is far less favourable for patients in whom there is an increased risk of seeding through the cerebrospinal fluid. In these cases, 5 year survival rates of 48% and 10 year survival rates of 35% have been achieved. Brain stem gliomas form a mixed group of tumours which are characterized by site rather than histological appearance. Survival figures are 30% at 5 years and 20% at 10 years. Suprasellar tumours which are rare, have been reported to have a 5 year disease-free survival of 60%.

SPINAL TUMOURS

Primary spinal tumours are very uncommon in childhood. The most common are the gliomas, which may be 'benign' (histological Grade I and II). Tumours that may metastasize to the spinal cord include primary brain tumours (medulloblastoma and ependymoma) and other primary tumours such as Ewing's sarcoma, lymphomas and leukaemia. Neuroblastoma may involve the spinal cord usually by direct extension through the intervertebral foramina, as with the classic 'dumbbell' lesion (Chapter 19).

In the case of primary spinal tumours, the development of paraplegia necessitates emergency action, namely a myelogram to determine site of block followed by emergency decompression laminectomy. In the case of metastatic tumours, there may be a case of deferring laminectomy and treating with chemotherapy and irradiation if toxic doses to the spinal cord have not been exceeded. A more insidious onset may occur with muscle weakness, muscle spasm, pain and abnormalities of sphincter control. Tumours of the cauda equina may present with low back pain and pain referred along the sciatic nerve. These symptoms may be mistaken for bony or intervertebral disc injuries. Diagnosis is confirmed by myelogram.

Standard treatment consists of surgery with removal of as much tumour as possible without damaging the cord. Postoperative irradiation therapy usually follows, the dose depending upon the age of the patient and the size of treatment field. A common regimen would be 35–40 Gy given over 4–5 weeks.

The role of chemotherapy in primary spinal tumours is unknown. Obviously, for secondary deposits such as neuroblastoma or lymphoma, chemotherapy will have a major role to play. The exact agents used depend upon the particular type of tumour.

RECOMMENDED READING

Bamford F.N., Morris-Jones P., Pearson D., Riberio G.G., Shalet S.M. & Beardwell C.G. (1976) Residual disabilities in children treated for intracranial space occupying lesions. *Cancer* **37**, 1149.

Cangir A., van Eys J., Berry D.H., Hvizdala E. & Morgan S.K. (1978) Combination chemotherapy with MOPP in children with recurrent brain tumours. *Medical and Pediatric Oncology* **4**, 253.

Cumberlin R.L., Luk K.H., Wara W.M., Sheline G.E. & Wilson C.B. (1979) Medulloblastoma. Treatment results and effect on normal tissues. *Cancer* **43**, 1014.

Dohrmann G.J., Farwell J.R. & Flannery J.T. (1976) Ependymomas and ependymoblastomas in children. *Journal of Neurosurgery* **45**, 273.

FARWELL J.R., DOHRMANN G.J. & FLANNERY J.T. (1977) Central nervous system tumours in children. *Cancer* **40**, 3123.

LEVIN V.A. & WILSON C.B. (1976) Nitrosourea chemotherapy for primary malignant gliomas. *Cancer Treatment Reports* **60**, 719.

TOKARS R.P., SUTTON H.G. & GRIEM M.L. (1979) Cerebellar medulloblastoma. Results of a new method of radiation treatment. *Cancer* **43**, 129.

WARA W.M., JENKIN R.D.T., EVANS A.E., ERTEL I., HITTLE R., ORTEGA J., WILSON C.B. & HAMMOND D. (1979) Tumours of the pineal and suprasellar region: Children's Cancer Study Group treatment results 1960–1975. *Cancer* **43**, 698.

Chapter 23
Miscellaneous Tumours

There are many unusual tumours in childhood, but they are rare, and it is outside the scope of this text to discuss their presentation and therapy in detail. Four of these tumours are, however, sufficiently frequent or associated with profound consequences to warrant description in some detail.

HISTIOCYTOSIS X

Pathology

This disease is peculiar to childhood and is characterized by proliferation of fixed tissue histiocytes associated with varying degrees of lymphocytic and eosinophilic infiltration and destruction of surrounding tissue. The exact nature of the disease is not well understood. It has many features of a malignant disorder with widespread involvement of the reticuloendothelial system by an infiltrative process, local tissue infiltration and dissemination. On the other hand, many forms of the disease behave in a benign manner; spontaneous fluctuations characterized by remissions and recurrences are sometimes seen; ill-defined immunological abnormalities have been described in association with it; and, most recently, some patients have responded to treatment with thymosine. This has led to the suggestion that at least some forms of histiocytosis X may be disorders of immune regulation.

On the basis of histological appearance, benign and malignant forms have been described. There is, however, very little association between the histological appearance and the eventual outcome of the disease or the response to treatment. The origin of the cells undergoing malignant transformation is unknown but, recently, it has been suggested that the distribution of the disease can be best accounted for if at least one of the cell groups involved are the fixed dermal and epithelial phagocytic cells, containing Langerhans cell granules. Some of the ultrastructural features of histiocytosis X cells and these cells are strikingly similar.

Clinical presentation

This seems to be related to the age at presentation. In children under the age of

2 years, there is often widespread involvement of skin, resulting in a salmon pink, seborrheic looking rash. The scalp and the skin behind the ears are most characteristically involved. Progression of the skin lesions may lead to superficial ulceration. In addition, there is frequently involvement of adjacent lymph nodes, liver and spleen. Destructive bone lesions are unusual in the youngest children, but may be present in those nearing the age of 2 years. This clinical picture has been given the eponymous name of Letterer-Siwe disease.

In children between the ages of 2 and 8 years, the disease usually presents with bone and soft tissue involvement, without widespread skin changes or infiltration of the reticuloendothelial system. Any bone in the body may be involved but, most frequently, there are destructive lesions of the petrous temporal together with otitis externa or mandibular and maxillary destructive lesions, with non-healing mouth ulcers. In these patients, there is often premature eruption of teeth. There is an association between skull and mouth lesions and the development of diabetes insipidus, which is presumably due to infiltration of the posterior pituitary. The constellation of symptoms in which there are destructive skull lesions and diabetes insipidus, has been given the eponymous name of Hand-Schüller-Christian disease.

In children above the age of 8 years, the disease usually presents with either single or multiple bone lesions without soft tissue involvement. Biopsy of these lesions reveals marked eosinophilic infiltration and, therefore, this condition has been called eosinophilic granuloma.

There are atypical presentations in all age groups; patients with characteristic features of the young and older age groups, and treated patients may revert from the type of presentation seen in infancy to that seen in the older age group. In all patients, the basic histological apearance is proliferation of tissue histiocytes. For these reasons, it is reasonable to consider this wide variety of clinical features as due to one disease process called histiocytosis X. Variations in the clinical picture are related to age as well as factors which are at present not known.

Investigations and staging

The diagnosis of histiocytosis X is confirmed by tissue biopsy of an involved organ, most commonly bone or skin. It is seldom necessary to excise a lymph node or perform a liver biopsy to establish the diagnosis. Staging depends upon demonstration of the extent of skeletal involvement by bone scan and/or skeletal survey, and by investigation of the presence or absence of organ dysfunction.

Organ dysfunction is assessed in the following way: *Bone marrow* by a full blood examination. Anaemia, neutropenia or thrombocytopenia not related to an intercurrent infection are considered to indicate bone marrow dysfunction. The presence of histiocytes in the marrow aspirate not associated with blood count abnormalities is not regarded as a sign of marrow dysfunction. *Liver dysfunction* is assessed by means of liver function studies and excretion of BSP. *Lung dysfunction* is assessed by means of chest radiogram and, whenever possible, pulmonary function studies. *Deafness* and *diabetes insipidus* secondary to histiocytosis X, are not regarded as organ dysfunction for the purposes of staging.

Patients without evidence of organ dysfunction are considered to have Stage I disease, and its severity can be assessed by the number of bones and organs infiltrated. The fewer the sites of infiltration, the better the prognosis. Patients with organ dysfunction have Stage II disease and have a worse prognosis than that of any patient with Stage I disease. In this group, there is no evidence of an association of prognosis with the number of bones or organs infiltrated with histiocytosis X.

Treatment

The need for treatment and the intensity of treatment depend upon the stage of the disease and the nature and number of organs involved.

Solitary bone lesions can usually be treated with surgical curettage and neither irradiation nor chemotherapy are required. However, solitary bone lesions may occur in critical places where surgical treatment is not possible, e.g. atlas or axis or femoral neck. In such patients, chemotherapy with cholorambucil 6 mg/m^2 has been very effective in accelerating bone healing. Chemotherapy is preferred to irradiation because of the long-term effects of irradiation on bone growth. Chlorambucil treatment is usually continued for 3–6 months depending on the rate of response and the extent of healing.

In patients with multiple bone lesions but no soft tissue involvement, or patients older than two years with bone and soft tissue involvement with Stage I disease, a response rate of 50–60% to chlorambucil therapy has been described, although subsequent reports indicate only a 27% response rate. In these patients, there is also a 20–30% relapse rate when chlorambucil is discontinued after 3 months of treatment. Although a second remission can usually be obtained with chlorambucil, it is arguable whether the long-term risks of prolonged chlorambucil treatment may not outweigh the discomfort of a Type II regimen. For these reasons, it is now common practice to commence patients with multiple bone lesions and soft tissue involvement or soft tissue involvement only, on combination chemotherapy.

The most extensive experience of combination chemotherapy has been obtained with a regimen proposed by Lahey and outlined below:

Vinblastine 6 mg/m^2 i.v. weekly × 8 on day 1
Prednisolone 40 mg/m^2 orally daily × 6 weeks, tapering during the last 2 weeks

Methotrexate 20 mg/m^2 orally or i.m. weekly × 8 on day 2
Cyclophosphamide 200 mg/m^2 orally x 8 on day 4.

After remission has been induced, maintenance chemotherapy consists of methotrexate and cyclophosphamide as above, with monthly booster doses of vinblastine given as two injections at one week intervals and prednisolone for one week. Chemotherapy is continued for 12–18 months. Prior to discontinuing treament, the patient should be investigated to ensure that there is no residual disease. Diabetes insipidus does not respond to treatment with chemotherapy or irradiation. It is controlled with pitressin or DDAVP and the use of these agents does not interfere with systemic chemotherapy. Combination chemotherapy in this disorder is immunosuppressive and in children who may already have a subtle immune deficiency, it is potentially hazardous. Particular attention must be paid to intercurrent infections and the use of long-term prophylactic Bactrim to prevent *Pneumocystis carinii* infections.

Prognosis

Five year disease-free rates for disseminated histiocytosis X vary from 50% to 80%. Progressive disease causing death is seen most often in children under the age of 1 year; in females with Stage II disease on presentation; or Stage II disease following relapse of Stage I disease.

In these patients, 2 year disease-free rates are approximately 30%. Some reports suggest that children with disseminated histiocytosis X may have stunting of growth and retarded mental development, but this has not been our experience.

HEPATIC TUMOURS

Incidence and pathology

Most hepatoblastomas occur in children under 3 years of age, predominantly in males. Hepatocarcinomas usually occur in older children. Hepatomas occur with increased frequency in both children and adults in Asia and Africa. The right lobe of the liver is more commonly affected than the left. Hepatocarcinomas arise more often in livers involved by a pre-existing disease, particularly cirrhosis. They tend to be multicentric and more invasive than hepatoblastomas which appear 'encapsulated' due to compression of normal liver tissue.

Microscopically in hepatoblastomas, epithelial cells predominate. In the mixed form, varying proportions of fetal mesenchymal tissue are seen. Hepatocarcinomas are indistinguishable from the adult carcinoma of the liver. Metastatic spread is usually regional and to the lungs, with bone and bone marrow rarely involved.

The clinical differential diagnosis is that of metastatic tumours of the liver and benign disorders. Neuroblastoma and Wilms' tumour are the most common tumours which metastasize to the liver. Lymph node involvement of porta hepatis nodes by lymphoma also needs to be considered. Appropriate investigations should be performed to exclude these disorders.

Haemangiomas, lymphangiomas and mesenchymal hamartoma are benign tumours of the liver which may have a similar clinical presentation to malignant neoplasms.

Investigations

Hepatic enlargement together with elevated levels of α-fetoproteins strongly suggest the diagnosis of hepatoblastoma. Radiological investigations such as ultrasound examination or CAT scans permit determination of the size and spread of tumour. Selective hepatic angiography may be required by surgeons if partial hepatectomy is contemplated. Plain X-rays of the chest, bone scans and bone marrow aspirations are required to stage the disease. The need for biopsy prior to definitive treatment is a matter of controversy. The presence of a hepatic mass, elevated levels of α-fetoproteins and metastatic disease may obviate the need for a surgical biopsy. On the other hand, if partial hepatectomy is to be undertaken, it is preferable to perform an open liver biopsy first and at a subsequent time, some days later, plan for the definitive procedure under deep hypothermia.

The level of α-fetoproteins is a useful means of following the progress of the disease. The level returns to normal 5–6 weeks after effective treatment of the primary. An elevation of α-fetoproteins should be considered as an early warning sign of primary recurrence or metastatic spread.

Treatment

Complete excision of the primary tumour, together with a wide margin of normal liver tissue, is the treatment of choice. Unless complete resection is achieved, cure is unlikely. There is now some evidence that initially inoperable primary tumours may be converted to operable tumours by the judicious use of intensive chemotherapy. Adriamycin is the most active agent, but vincristine, 5-fluorouracil and cyclophosphamide also have some activity. The four agents are usually used in combination. Irradiation therapy has little role, if any, to play in the treatment of primary liver tumours of childhood.

Prognosis

The prognosis depends entirely on whether the primary tumour is operable or not. If so, a 75% cure rate can be expected. Few, if any, cures can be expected in patients with residual or metastatic disease despite the use of chemotherapy, but useful palliation may be achieved.

GERM CELL TUMOURS

Embryology

Germ cells appear at an early stage of development and are initially located in the wall of the yolk sac close to the allantois. From there, they migrate towards the region of the genital ridges. In the sixth week of development, the germ cells invade the genital ridges. Their migration into these ridges has an inductive effect on the development of the gonads. The interaction of the germ cells, epithelium and mesenchyme eventually result in the formation of mature testes or ovary. The characteristics of germ cell tumours can be best understood by bearing in mind the pluripotential nature of these cells and their migratory characteristic.

Five distinct neoplasms may arise from these tumours: (1) Seminoma, (2) embryonal carcinoma, (3) teratoma, (4) chorioncarcinoma and (5) yolk sac tumours. Some of these neoplasms show more than one histological pattern, while, in others, there is only one component. In paediatrics, the teratomas, embryonal carcinomas and yolk sac tumours are more important than seminomas and chorioncarcinomas, which are predominantly tumours of the adult years.

Teratomas

They occur in a variety of sites, most commonly midline and gonadal. They may present in the neonatal period, infancy or childhood, and may be benign or malignant, solid or cystic. The most common site is the sacrococcygeal region, but they may also be found in the retroperitoneum, mediastinum and base of skull.

SACROCOCCYGEAL

Sacrococcygeal teratomas account for 60–70% of teratomas. They most commonly present at birth when they cause difficult labour. In such patients, the swelling is obvious. In later months, the tumour may present with symptoms due to local extension such as constipation, urinary obstruction, failure to walk or an obvious pelvic or gluteal mass. Histologically, the tumour contains tissues arising from all three embryonic layers. If malignant transformation has occurred, then it is predominantly of the yolk cell carcinoma type. The α-fetoproteins level is frequently raised, and this serves as a useful diagnostic tool as well as allowing serial measurements of the response of the tumour to therapy. The incidence of malignancy is related to age, with approximately 6% being malignant before six months of age and 50–60% malignant beyond this age. The differential diagnosis is that of meningocoele, haemangioma, lymphangioma, chordoma or neurogenic tumour.

TREATMENT

Benign tumours can usually be excised totally with the coccyx. Malignant tumours tend to extend by local infiltration. Metastases occur most commonly to bones and/or lungs. Despite surgical excision, the prognosis is uniformly poor.

Classically malignant sacrococcygeal teratomas are stated to be insensitive to irradiation and chemotherapy.

Recent experience with combination chemotherapy and the development of treatment regimens containing *cis*-platinum have changed the poor prognosis of patients with these tumours. In tumours that are not excisable, a needle biopsy may establish the diagnosis, following which intensive chemotherapy should be administered to shrink the tumour and make it surgically resectable. Chemotherapy regimens usually consist of vincristine, cyclophosphamide, actinomycin D and adriamycin. As an alternative, VAB regimens consisting of vinblastine, actinomycin D, bleomycin and *cis*-platinum, may be used. The difficulties of monitoring *cis*-platinum in young children make VAB therapy unattractive and it should probably be reserved for patients failing to respond to other drug combinations, or older than 8 years at the time of presentation. Following one or two courses of chemotherapy, marked tumour regression usually occurs, making surgical excision with a wide margin of normal tissues a possibility. Depending upon the age of the child and the surgical findings, postoperative irradiation to the tumour bed may also be used. Chemotherapy is continued for 18 months to 2 years.

The previously poor prognosis ($\simeq$ 30% survival) of malignant tumours will undoubtedly be improved by the above approach.

Ovarian

Ovarian tumours in children are predominantly of germ cell type with dysgerminoma, embryonal (endodermal sinus) carcinoma and malignant teratoma. They are rare tumours, constituting less than 2% of paediatric solid tumours. The usual modes of presentation are with abdominal swelling associated with pressure on surrounding sites, torsion, haemorrhage or rupture of cyst, all of which are associated with sudden, severe abdominal pain often accompanied by shock. Ascites is a rare presentation.

The diagnosis is usually suspected on clinical grounds and the ovarian origin of the tumours is established by ultrasound or CAT scans. Staging of the tumour should be performed by non-surgical means such as an isotope bone scan, lymphangiography and CAT scans of lungs. The α-fetoproteins may be elevated and serve as a useful marker of the response of tumour to treatment.

Treatment consists of total surgical removal of the tumour. In the case of large dysgerminomas and teratomas, hysterectomy and bilateral salpingo-oöphorectomy are recommended. In embryonal yolk sac carcinoma, there is no evidence that hysterectomy and bilateral salpingo-oöphorectomy improve the prognosis. Because of the propensity of these tumours to metastasize, combination chemotherapy as described for the teratomas should be used. Irradiation to pelvis and involved lymph node areas is reserved for dysgerminomas or mixed tumours in which dysgerminoma is the predominant element.

Testicular

As in ovarian tumours, the majority of testicular tumours are of germ cell origin. Their incidence peaks in infancy and falls to extremely low levels between 3 years of age and puberty. Three main types of tumour are seen: (1) Embryonal adenocarcinoma; also called orchioblastoma, endodermal sinus tumour, Teilum's tumour, and adenocarcinoma with clear cells; (2) embryonal carcinoma; and (3) teratocarcinoma.

The tumours usually present as a local swelling which may be associated with a hydrocoele. Occasionally, torsion of the testes may be a presenting feature. Rarely, teratocarcinomas secreting chorionic gonadotrophins may produce symptoms of precocious puberty.

The diagnosis is suggested by the presence of a firm testicular mass and, in the case of embryonal adenocarcinomas, a markedly elevated level of α-fetoproteins. Biopsy confirms the diagnosis and should be excisional if clinical findings and frozen section confirm malignancy. Lymphangiography and CAT scans of abdomen and lungs are required to stage the disease. Embryonal adenocarcinomas which have not metastasized can usually be successfully treated with surgery alone. Monitoring of the response of the tumour with α-fetoprotein levels is continued for 2 years. In embryonal carcinomas and teratocarcinomas, Stage I lesions are treated by radical orchiectomy and by retroperitoneal lymph node dissection. If lymph nodes are not involved, further therapy may be withheld.

In children with any one of the three types of tumour and metastatic disease to lymph nodes or distal sites, intensive chemotherapy may produce resolution of disease. As in teratomas in children under the age of 8 years, combinations of vincristine, adriamycin, actinomycin D and cyclophosphamide are effective. In older children, vinblastine, actinomycin D, bleomycin and *cis*-platinum are preferred.

RETINOBLASTOMA

Incidence

This is a rare tumour occurring in one in 23 000 births. Because of its effect on vision and its hereditary nature, its importance far outweighs its numerical incidence. The diagnosis is usually made before 2 years of age and often in early infancy. Early diagnosis markedly improves the prognosis of this tumour. Approximately two-thirds of retinoblastomas are unilateral. About 5% of patients who initially present with unilateral disease subsequently show tumour foci in the opposite retina.

Hereditary pattern

There have been sufficient survivors over a number of generations in this tumour to permit accurate observations on its inheritance. A pattern of dominant inheritance in families with bilateral retinoblastoma has been known for many years, while in patients with unilateral retinoblastoma, transmission of the disease to offspring is much less common. Affected offspring of patients with unilateral or bilateral retinoblastoma often have bilateral tumours suggesting that the same gene may be involved in hereditary unilateral and bilateral retinoblastomas. Knudson has developed a model to explain these findings. He suggested that all retinoblastomas might result from two mutations. In the hereditary form, the first mutation occurs in a germ cell line and thus the genetic information is present in all cells of the embryo. A single second event may then lead to the development of cancer. Such tumours would occur early in life and could be multiple. The findings of a 10% occurrence of second tumours in children with bilateral retinoblastomas fits well with Knudson's model.

In non-hereditary cases, the same two events would be necessary in the same somatic cell line. The probability of this happening is so low that such tumours would almost always be single.

Gene carriers of the germinal mutation might develop no tumours, single tumours or multiple tumours, depending on the frequency of second mutations.

On the basis of Knudson's model, all bilateral and 20% of unilateral retinoblastomas could be attributed to a hereditary origin.

Retinoblastoma occasionally occurs in children with multiple congenital abnormalities associated with deletion of a part of the long arm of Group 13 chromosomes. Banding techniques show that Band 14 of Group 13 chromosome may be the site of the genes for retinoblastoma. Recently, esterase D has been found to be associated with the same band and it is hoped that it may serve as a biochemical marker for that type of retinoblastoma.

The following guidelines for genetic counselling in this tumour can be obtained from large multi-generations studies:

1 Identifiable gene carriers (bilateral or familial retinoblastoma; family history of retinoblastoma and affected offspring; evidence of spontaneous regression): risk in offspring 50%. Affected offspring have 70% chance of bilateral tumours and 10% chance of other cancers.

2 Unilateral retinoblastoma with no family history: risk to subsequent sibling 3%. Risk to offspring of the affected individual 7–10%.

3 Bilateral retinoblastoma with no family history: risk to subsequent sibling 10–20%. Risks to offspring of the affected individual 50%.

4 Risk to offspring of an unaffected sibling of a patient with retinoblastoma is low, but some authorities recommend ophthalmic examination under general anaesthesia.

Pathology

Histologically, the tumour shows undifferentiated small round cells with deeply staining nuclei and scant cytoplasm. Larger cells that form rosettes around a central cavity are also seen. The tumour is multifocal in the majority of patients. Seeding in large tumours may occur into the vitreous or the tumour may grow into the sub-retinal space causing retinal detachment. Extension of tumour into the choroid layer occurs with large tumours, but does not necessarily indicate that haematogenous metastases will occur. The most dangerous extensions are those along the optic nerve. If the tumour extends 10–12 mm along the nerve to the point where the central retinal artery and vein enter and leave the nerve, then there is a high probability of base of skull and meningeal seeding by the tumour.

Clinical features

Early tumours are seldom symptomatic and are diagnosed only if there is a family history of retinoblastoma and there are regular eye examinations. Usually, the tumour presents because the parents notice a white pupil — 'cat's eye reflex'. Strabismus and red and painful eye with or without glaucoma are the next most common presenting features. Fortunately, proptosis and fungating tumours are nowadays exceedingly rare.

Examination of the eye is usually undertaken under general anaesthesia with indirect ophthalmoscopy. A number of appearances have been described ranging from obvious fungating tumour to retinal detachment. The details of ophthalmic appearances of the tumour should be sought in appropriate opthalmological texts. The local extent of the tumour can be assessed by CAT scans. The cerebrospinal fluid should be examined for tumour cells and radioisotope bone scan, plain chest X-rays and bone marrow aspiration performed to stage the tumour.

Ophthalmological examination frequently cannot establish the diagnosis of retinoblastoma with certainty. The differential diagnoses include parasitic infestations, vascular malformations, congenital retinal defects and retinal detachment. Confirmation of diagnosis should be pursued by an experienced ophthalmologist, preferably in an oncology centre. Extensive disease will usually require enucleation of the eye, irrespective of diagnosis as vision has been lost in the affected eye. In bilateral disease, the most extensively involved eye is enucleated. In patients with unilateral disease, no family history of retinoblastoma and lesions which do not destroy vision, frequent observation of the appearance of the tumour by an experienced opthalmologist is reasonable until a decision can be made on the nature of the lesion.

Staging of disease

The staging system given in Table 23.1 has been devised by Rees and collaborators, and by Ellsworth. The prognosis refers to chance of preservation of vision, not survival. Staging is accomplished by exact diagrammatic and photographic location of all tumours.

Treatment

SURGERY

In unilateral retinoblastoma with extensive disease (Groups IV and V), the involved eye is enucleated. In bilateral disease, the more extensively involved is enucleated if there is little chance of preserving vision in that eye. Occasionally, in bilateral retinoblastomas with very extensive disease in both eyes (Group V), bilateral enucleation is preferred. When enucleation is undertaken, as much of the optic nerve as possible should also be removed, since tumour extension beyond the point where the retinal vessels enter suggests that there may be involvement of the subarachnoid space. Following enucleation, it is essential to fit an early prosthesis and to continue changing the prosthesis as the child grows. In case of bilateral enucleation, contact should be established with societies which care for and educate the blind, so that rehabilitation can start as soon as feasible.

Table 23.1 Staging system for retinoblastoma.

Group I Very favourable	
1	Solitary tumours, less than 4 disc diameters in size, at or behind the equator
2	Multiple tumours, none over 4 disc diameters in size, all at or behind equator
Group II Favourable	
1	Solitary lesion, 4–10 disc diameters in size, at or behind the equator
2	Multiple tumours, 4–10 disc diameters in size, behind the equator
Group III Doubtful	
1	Any lesion anterior to the equator
2	Solitary tumours larger than 10 disc diameters behind the equator
Group IV Unfavourable	
1	Multiple tumours, some larger than 10 disc diameters
2	Any lesion extending anteriorly to the ora serrata
Group V Very unfavourable	
1	Massive tumours involving over half the retina
2	Vitreous seeding

IRRADIATION

This is the mainstay of treatment of Group I, II and III lesions. The precise fields of irradiation must be carefully defined on the basis of existing disease. Irradiation should be administered only in centres with experience in the treatment of this tumour. Megavoltage therapy is used and appropriate fields are constructed to encompass all tumour. As a minimum, the entire retina posterior to the equator should be included. In Groups I, II and III, the dose to the retina is 35 Gy in 3 weeks. In Groups IV and V tumours, the dose is 45 Gy in 4 weeks.

In the case of confirmed extension of the tumour outside the globe of the eye or lesions of the optic nerve, the orbital fossa should be irradiated after enucleation. If, on CAT scan and/or examination of the CSF, there is evidence of tumour extension into the base of skull or the subarachnoid space, craniospinal irradiation to 24 Gy may be used as a means of controlling the disease. Unfortunately, such treatment is seldom successful in eradicating CNS retinoblastoma.

In some centres, radioactive applicators are used. This is reserved for tumours with extension to the choroid, residual tumours too large for light coagulation or small tumours located posteriorly or at the ora serrata. The use of these applicators is again limited to centres which have gained expertise in this technique.

LIGHT COAGULATION

This is of particular use in tumours anterior to the equator that do not show satisfactory tumour shrinkage 4–6 weeks after irradiation. It is also of use in the treatment of recurrent retinoblastoma. Tumours up to 4 disc diameter well removed from the optic nerve are particularly suitable for light coagulation.

CHEMOTHERAPY

The mortality rate in retinoblastomas is 18%. Approximately half the patients die of metastatic disease to bone and lungs, and the other half of metastatic disease to the central nervous system. Mortality figures greater than 50% are seen in Group V patients, those with extensions to the orbit or those presenting with disseminated disease. Initially, intra-arterial triethylenemelamine was used as a single agent, but subsequently it has been shown that combination chemotherapy with vincristine, cyclophosphamide and adriamycin can be very effective. The use of chemotherapy is usually restricted to patients with Group V disease, orbital extensions or disseminated disease. In patients with extensions to the central nervous system, in addition to craniospinal irradiation, monthly intrathecal methotrexate has been used. The value of such treatment is difficult to determine at the present time.

Prognosis

The following data given in Table 23.2 has been reported from the Columbia-Presbyterian Medical Center in a review of 192 patients with bilateral disease treated between 1960–65. Control rate refers to preservation of vision and survival. Minimal follow-up was 3 years.

In patients with bilateral retinoblastoma, there is also a 10% incidence of second tumours which may occur at, or distant from, the site of irradiation. These tumours include osteosarcomas, lymphomas and leukaemia.

LONG-TERM SEQUELAE OF TREATMENT

Impairment of vision through irradiation is kept to a minimum if doses do not exceed 50 Gy. Cataracts also occur rarely when proper megavoltage irradiation is given. Irradiation may interfere with bone growth and occasionally there is damage to the pituitary, leading to hypopituitarism.

Table 23.2 Review of 192 patients with bilateral retinoblastoma.

Group	Number of patients	Control rate (%)
I	20	95
II	32	87
III	24	67
IV	32	69
V	74	34
Orbital	10	30

RECOMMENDED READING

Histiocytosis X

Komp D.M., Vietti T.J., Berry B.H., Starling K.A., Haggard M.E. & George S.L. (1977) Combination chemotherapy in histiocytosis X. *Medical and Pediatric Oncology* **3**, 267.

Lahey M.E. (1975) Histiocytosis X. Treatment regimens. *Journal of Pediatrics* **87**, 179.

Lahey M.E. (1975) Histiocytosis X. Prognostic factors. *Journal of Pediatrics* **87**, 184.

Lichtenstein L. (1964) Histiocytosis X (eosinophilic granuloma of bone, Letterer-Siwe disease and Schuller-Christian disease). Further observations of pathological and clinical importance. *Journal of Bone and Joint Surgery* **46**, 76.

Smith P.J., Ekert H. & Campbell P.E. (1976) Improved prognosis in disseminated histiocytosis. *Medical and Pediatric Oncology* **2**, 371.

Toogood I.R.G., Ellis W.M. & Ekert H. (1979) Prognostic criteria, treatment and survival in disseminated histiocytosis X. *Australian Paediatric Journal* **15**, 91.

Hepatic tumours

HOLTON C.P., BURRINGTON J.D. & HATCH E.I. (1975) A multiple chemotherapeutic approach to the management of hepatoblastoma. *Cancer* **35**, 1083.

SIEGEL M.M., SIEGEL S.E., ISAACS H., WEITZMAN J.J., HANSON B.A., HIGGINS G.R. & SHORE N.A. (1978) Primary chemotherapeutic management of unresectable and metastatic hepatoblastoma in children. *Medical and Pediatric Oncology* **4**, 297.

Germ cell tumours

CANGIR A., SMITH J., & VAN EYS J. (1978) Improved prognosis in children with ovarian cancers following modified VAC (vincristine sulfate, dactinomycin and cyclophosphamide) chemotherapy. *Cancer* **42**, 1234.

EXELBY P. (1979) Testis cancer in children. *Seminars in Oncology* **VI**, 116.

GROSFIELD J.L., BALLANTINE T.J., LOWE D. & BAEHNER R.L. (1976) Benign and malignant teratomas in children: analysis of 85 patients. *Surgery* **80**, 297.

SUTOW W.W., VIETTI T.J. & FERNBACH D.J. (1973) *Clinical Pediatric Oncology*, pp. 515, 562. C.V. Mosby, St Louis.

YORBO J.W. (ed.) (1979) Germ cell tumours. *Seminars in Oncology* **VI**, 1.

Retinoblastoma

ELLSWORTH R.M. (1969) The practical management of retinoblastoma. *Transactions of The American Opthalmologic Society* **67**, 462.

JENSEN R.D. & MILLER R.W. (1971) Retinoblastoma: epidemiologic characteristics. *New England Journal of Medicine* **285**, 307.

KNUDSON A.G.J. (1971) Mutation and cancer: A statistical study of retinoblastoma. *Proceedings of the National Academy of Sciences, USA* **68**, 820.

REESE A.B., HYMAN G.A., MERRIAM JR G.R., FORREST A.W. & KLIGERMAN M.M. (1955) Treatment of retinoblastoma by radiation and triethylenemelamine. *Archives of Ophthalmology* **53**, 505.

SPARKES R.S., SPARKES M.C., WILSON M.G., TOWNER J.W., BENEDICT W., MURPHREE A.L. & YUNIS J.J. (1980) Regional assignment of genes for human esterase D and retinoblastoma to chromosome band 13914. *Science* **208**, 1042.

STRONG L.C. (1977) Genetic considerations in pediatric oncology. In *Clinical Pediatric Oncology* (eds W.W. SUTOW, T.J. VIETTI & D.J. FERNBACH). C.V. Mosby, St Louis.

TAPLEY DU V. N. (1977) Retinoblastoma. In *Clinical Pediatric Oncology* (eds. W.W. SUTOW, T.J. VIETTI & D.J. FERNBACH). C.V. Mosby, St Louis.

Index